CW00447618

Index

7- *Mushroom frittata with goat cheese*
8- *Ketogenic veggie scramble*
9- *Delicious Ketogenic taco omelet.*
10- *Basil and butter scramble with eggs.*

B- Ketogenic lunch recipes.

- **Non-vegetarian**

1- *Ketogenic paleo baked meatballs.*
2- *Low carb dairy-free butter chicken.*
3- *Ketogenic fat-head pizza.*
4- *Keto Tortilla Española.*
5- *Special ketogenic Lamb kofta kebabs*

- **Vegetarian**

1- *Low carb taco salad.*
2- *Salmon, Avocado and Arugula Salad.*
3- *Fennel and Celery Salad.*
4- *Keto Cauliflower Rice Salad*
5- *Ketogenic cauliflower potato salad.*

C- Special Ketogenic Dinner.

- ***Non-vegetarian***

1- *Creamy Tuscan garlic chicken.*
2- *Keto grilled Mediterranean chicken salad.*

3- Cauliflower rice with chicken meatballs.
4- Tasty Keto zucchini slice.
5- Ketogenic pan-seared steaks with mushrooms.

- **Vegetarian**

1- Keto Broccoli Cheddar Soup.
2- Cheese shell taco cups.
3- Gluten-Free Cheese and Cauliflower 'Breadsticks'
4- Low-Carb Lasagna Stuffed Spaghetti Squash.
5- Keto vegan Sushi Bowl.

D- Ketogenic Dessert recipes.

1- Keto chocolate mug cake.
2- Ketogenic ice cream.
3- Keto peanut chocolate blocks.
4- Low carb walnut snow balls.
5- Ketogenic brownies.

Author's Notes

It's Antonio Tagliafierro, the author of this cook book. This is not just a cook book but is also my life experience. You may call it just a simple cook book, but it is a book that contains inspiration and motivation for many lives. During writing this book, I was more concerned about the lives that are going to get benefit from it rather than the recipes and their tastes. You can bring taste in a recipe by adding or skipping few ingredients but bringing taste in the life of someone is the real art.

We all know that obesity and heavy weight has become a global health problem. A lot of people die of this disease every year and others who live also face a lot of difficulties. They are not just facing physical difficulties but also psychological difficulties stand in their way. They bear criticism from people for their heavy weight. People would make fun out of them without caring for their feelings. And as a result, they become psychologically disturbed as well. And a human who is already physically disturbed, becomes psychologically disturbed then what is left in his or her life.

This is what I experienced in my life. I weighed 140 kg and I faced the similar physical and psychological problems. But instead of giving up in front of this world, I packed myself up and decided to lose weight and to show my mental strength to people around me. I decided that I will one day lose my weight and not only lose my own weight but will also become a kind of inspiration for other people suffering from same problems as well. I took a stand and I started my journey!

I want to mention one more thing that I am a professional chef. And I already knew many kinds of diets and I often tried a lot. But the results were not satisfactory in terms of health and in terms of taste as well. Who can judge taste better than a chief!

Then I happened to learn about ketogenic diet. I had much knowledge about this type of diet already but there were some myths related to this diet like it causes brain diseases, it caused people to die etc. So I used to ignore Ketogenic diet. But then, after trying many options when nothing happened, I decided to study the one remaining option and that was "Ketogenic Diet".

I started following Ketogenic diet and as a chief prepared a lot of recipes that really helped me out more than any kind of diet and I got the best results. From 140 kg, I dropped to 80 kg after following Keto diet! You may get shocked by the results but it is my personal experience!

Ketogenic diet is basically a habit of healthy diet. You just need to leave high carbs meals and drinks and here you are in a journey towards losing your weight and enjoying your life!

The recipes that are given in this book are not just recipes, these are medicines that I used to lose weight and now I want to prescribe these medicines to my dear readers who are curious about losing weight but are not getting results so far.

Beauty of this book lies in a fact that it contains recipes that are not only healthier but are also tastier! These recipes will not taste less than any normal day diet or meal! Just try these easy recipes, satisfy your taste buds and also lose your weight!

You need not to worry about your heavy weight when you have got this cook book in your hands. You just need to go to the kitchen and bang!!

Author,

Antonio Tagliafierro

Ketogenic diet an introduction

The word **"Ketogenic"** means a diet with low-carb content (like the Atkins diet). In this type of diet, body gets calories from proteins and fats instead of carbohydrates.

This is very low carb and high fats diet and is a lot similar to Atkins and other low carb diets. The main idea of ketogenic diet is to reduce the intake of carbohydrates and replace most of the carbs with fats. This reduction in carbohydrates intake starts a metabolic activity called "ketosis" in the body. This diet got its name by this "ketosis" process.

In this metabolic state, the body efficiently burns fat for energy. It is also good for brain as it also converts fat into ketones in lever that transfer energy to brain.

In ketogenic diet, the foods we mostly eat contain **55% to 60% fat, 30% to 35% protein and 5% to 10% carbohydrates**.

Origin of ketogenic diet:

Historically speaking, Russell Wilder in 1921 first used the ketogenic diet to treat epilepsy. For more than 10 years the ketogenic diet was used as a medical treatment for pediatric epilepsy. But with the passage of time, the idea started to build to use the ketogenic diet as a rapid weight loss formula. In present days, ketogenic diet is more popular as a weight losing formula as compared to a medical treatment. But yes! Weight loss is not less than a medical treatment as well.

Types of ketogenic diet:

Ketogenic diet evolved through medical and scientific processes. The experts have categorized the ketogenic diet into 4 types.

1- **Standard Ketogenic diet (SKD) :**
   This is a high fat diet with moderate protein content and very low carb content. It contains 70 % fat, 20 % protein and 10 % carbs.

2- **Cyclical ketogenic diet (CKD):**
   This is a periodic type diet plan. It comprises of periods of low carb fee and high carb refeeds. For example, a 7 day cyclical diet plan means 5 days ketogenic days with low carb intake followed by 2 days with high carb intake.

3- **Targeted ketogenic diet (TKD):**
   This diet allows you to add carbs during workout or exercise.

4- **High protein ketogenic diet:**
   Just like standard ketogenic diet, this is low carb diet. But protein content is more than SKD. The ratio is often 60 % fat, 35 % protein and 5 % carbs.

However, only the standard and high protein ketogenic diets have been studied comprehensively. The other two types are considered more advanced methods and are used by body builders or athletes etc.

Health Benefits of ketogenic diet: A tasty medicine

Weight loss:

The medical sciences have advanced a lot but there still remain some challenges. Obesity is one of the greatest challenges that stand in front of the medical sciences. Obesity continue to remain a worldwide health problem and a challenge with adult mortality as high as 2.8 million per year. Obesity is not a single disease but it invites a lot of other chronic diseases as well. The diseases like diabetes, hypertension and heart diseases are largely related to obesity. Obesity is mainly caused due to unhealthy life style and poor dietary habits and routines.

Ketogenic diet has brought a hope for people suffering from obesity. It is for sure not the ultimate cure for the disease but can reduce the weight up to a large extent. And if an individual puts some more effort than surely this diet can be proven as the desired cure for the obesity.

The prime purpose and benefit of ketogenic diet is weight loss. Studies found that ketogenic diet was more effective than a low-fat diet for weight loss. But ketogenic diet is not confined to just weight loss; there are other health benefits as well.

 Studies found that people following ketogenic diet are less exposed to diabetes or pre-diabetes. Keto diet boosts the insulin sensitivity and burns fat. It is also found that type 2 diabetic patients have decreased level of diabetes after following ketogenic diet. Ketogenic diet causes reduction in seizures in epilepsy. It is also beneficial and is kinds of tasty cure for heart diseases, cancer, Parkinson's disease, polycystic ovary syndrome and brain diseases.

The science of ketogenic diet

How does keto diet work?

Basically, carbohydrates are the primary source of energy production in body tissues. When the body is deprived of carbohydrates due to reducing intake to less than 50g per day, insulin secretion is significantly reduced and the body enters a catabolic state. Glycogen stores deplete, forcing the body to go through certain metabolic changes. Two metabolic processes come into action when there is low carbohydrate availability in body tissues: gluconeogenesis and ketogenesis.

Gluconeogenesis is the endogenous production of glucose in the body, especially in the liver primarily from lactic acid, glycerol, and the amino acids alanine and glutamine. When glucose availability drops further, the endogenous production of glucose is not able to keep up with the needs of the body and ketogenesis begins in order to provide an alternate source of energy in the form of ketone bodies. Ketone bodies replace glucose as a primary source of energy. During ketogenesis due to low blood glucose feedback, stimulus for insulin secretion is also low, which sharply reduces the stimulus for fat and glucose storage. Other hormonal changes may contribute to the increased breakdown of fats that result in fatty acids. Fatty acids are metabolized to acetoacetate which is later converted to beta-hydroxybutyrate and acetone. These are the basic ketone bodies that accumulate in the body as a ketogenic diet is sustained. This metabolic state is referred to as "nutritional ketosis." As long as the body is deprived of carbohydrates, metabolism remains in the ketotic state. The nutritional ketosis state is considered quite safe, as ketone bodies are produced in small concentrations without any alterations in blood pH. It greatly differs from ketoacidosis, a life-threatening condition where ketone bodies are produced in extremely larger concentrations, altering blood pH to acidotic a state.

Ketone bodies synthesized in the body can be easily utilized for energy production by heart, muscle tissue, and the kidneys. Ketone bodies also can cross the blood-brain barrier to provide an alternative source of energy to the brain. RBCs and the liver do not utilize ketones due to lack of mitochondria and enzyme diaphoresis respectively. Ketone body production depends on several factors such as resting basal metabolic rate (BMR), body mass index (BMI), and body fat percentage. One hundred grams of acetoacetate generates 9400 grams of ATP, and 100 g of beta-hydroxybutyrate yields 10,500 grams of ATP; whereas, 100 grams of glucose produces only 8,700 grams of ATP. This allows the body to maintain efficient fuel production even during a caloric deficit. Ketone bodies also decrease free radical damage and enhance antioxidant capacity.

Summary:

On a simple and short note, ketogenic diet works as an alternative of glucose. Human body experiences two processes to get energy. First is gluconeogenesis, in this process body tissues and muscles use glucose as a source which is mainly produced in the liver. When carbs intake is reduced the production of glucose decreases. As a result body starts finding an alternative to get energy. It is the time when another process 'ketogenesis' starts. In ketogenesis, body starts getting energy from fats and as a result body fat burns and man starts losing weight.

Important questions and their answers

1- Who can and cannot follow the keto diet?

It is not necessary that only people suffering from obesity can follow the keto diet, this diet for everyone as it is healthier and energetic. So anyone who is willing can follow the diet.

Yet there are some people who cannot follow the ketogenic diet plan because of some diseases. People suffering from diabetes and taking insulin or oral hypoglycemic agents suffer severe hypoglycemia if the medications are not appropriately adjusted before initiating this diet. The ketogenic diet is contraindicated in patients with pancreatitis, liver failure, disorders of fat metabolism, primary carnitine deficiency, carnitine palmitoyl transferase deficiency, carnitine translocase deficiency, porphyria, or pyruvate kinase deficiency. People on a ketogenic diet rarely can have a false positive breath alcohol test. Due to ketonemia, acetone in the body can sometimes be reduced to isopropanol by hepatic alcohol dehydrogenase which can give a false positive alcohol breath test result.

2- Does it cost too much to follow ketogenic diet?

Well, that's not a case. Even if it cost a bit, would you ignore its medicinal benefits? But still it doesn't cost any extra money and in some cases it is less expensive than normal day diets. Moreover, it saves your pocket because you stop spending your earnings on fast foods and junk foods. You also leave most of the cold drinks and juices that are high carb and as a result this diet proves to be a very budget friendly and even a budget helping diet.

The ingredients and tools that are mostly used to prepare ketogenic meal are less expensive and are mostly available at home or local market. Most of the vegetables used are not so expensive. Sometimes you need to use olive oil or avocado oil for cooking and frying purposes, these type of ingredients may cost you a little. Use of mozzarella cheese and cream cheese also adds up in cost and often makes the diet expensive but still, one is not going to eat cheesy meal daily so you need not to worry about the cost. It is completely budget friendly and in some cases if it is costly, than remember its health benefits.

The recipes that are discussed in this book are moderate. There are some recipes that may be a little costly but there are also some recipes that will not cost you a lot. So, this book is a complete package containing basic, standard and premier recipes so that people may decide to choose a recipe according to their pocket.

3- Is it harmful for body?

It is not harmful for body if is done within limits prescribed by medical experts. It is universal truth that excess of anything is poisonous. Same is the matter in this case. If ketogenic diets are taken for a much longer time, the glucose will decrease to a vulnerable amount in body. As a result, the ketogenesis will start increasing acidity in the blood. That's why it is advised to follow ketogenic diet in form of a short term plan.

4- What to eat and what avoid during keto diet:

So that is the most common question that comes in minds of most of the people while talking about ketogenic diet. Everyone doesn't have a laboratory at home to test which ingredients are high carb and which one is low carb. So, let's see, what things we have to avoid during the keto diet.

> ➢ First of all, forget the fast and junk food! You cannot go near to it if you are following a keteo plan.
> ➢ Secondly, consider the drinks your worst enemies. The drinks are one of the biggest cause of obesity worldwide. So keep yourself away from this poison.
> ➢ Thirdly, you will need to leave few things that you love a lot, surely you are

not going to leave your wife or husband but yes! You will need to leave bread, sugar, starches and sometimes potatoes also. It means no more fries, no more crispy potato chips. But you've got some best dishes in ketogenic menu that will make you forget fries and fast food. So, you need not to worry much!

➤ One more a vastly used thing that you are going to leave is cooked rice. But there is an alternative for it. You can enjoy the taste of rice in shape of cauliflower rice and the cauliflower recipes are also included in the recipe list.

Other than these, you can use almost all the ingredients you like.

So, that was all about understanding ketogenic diet. Now! It's time to start following and preparing the diet in a delicious way. Let's get into the kitchen of keto diet and reduce weight with a tasty medicine!

Ketogenic Breakfast recipes

If you're following a ketogenic diet, you know you have to start paying attention to your carb intake from the moment you wake up and cook up your usual groggy-eyed breakfast. The keto diet is essentially a lower carb version of a low-carb diet. It doesn't count calories, but keeps a very watchful eye on the macros you consume every day. While the total amount varies from person to person, the ketogenic diet aims to limit total carbs to about 20 grams a day, while also eating a moderate amount of protein and lots of fats. The goal is getting into a state of ketosis, where your body burns fat rather than carbs for fuel.

When someone hears about diet, the first thing that comes in mind is 'salad' and sometimes a lot of 'salad'. Most of the people think that only salad is allowed during diet plan but it is not true. Ketogenic diet is a comprehensive diet plan. You can cook the breakfast, lunch and dinner according to your choice but you will need to follow the limits and ingredients of ketogenic diet to prepare your food. When you start following a ketogenic diet plan basically you start learning how to make the meals you love in some other alternative ways using different ingredients. The basic difference between your normal day meal and keto meal is the use of ingredients. You shift yourself from high carb to low carb ingredients. Some of the best ketogenic recipes to try in the breakfast are discussed below.

1- Keto egg muffins:

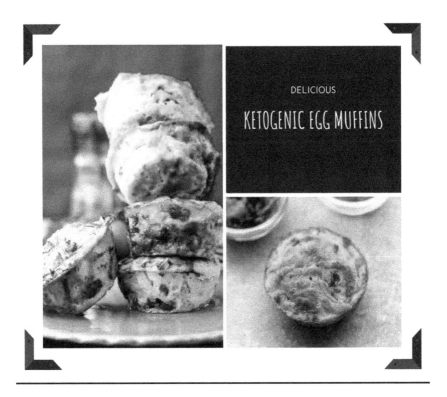

The low carb and high fats breakfast with an unbeatable taste and is easier to make as well, what else do you need if you have keto egg muffins recipe? Whether you're on a low carb or Keto diet, or you need something quick to grab while running out of the door, Breakfast Egg Muffins are a delicious healthy savior and perfect for Meal Prep!

There are some people who would not consider a morning a real morning if the breakfast table lacks a plate with eggs. They consider the egg as important to start the morning as coffee or tea. Keto egg muffins is a kind of keto package for egg lovers.

The easier to make, the tastier to eat. This dish can be cooked in 30-40 minutes but the taste doesn't leave the tongue whole day. It is one of the best, easiest and tastiest keto foods. These loaded, protein-packed egg muffins are for anyone who loves the satisfying combination of cheesy eggs. As you make the muffins, each cup will seem quite full with the cheddar filling. That's exactly how it's supposed to look.

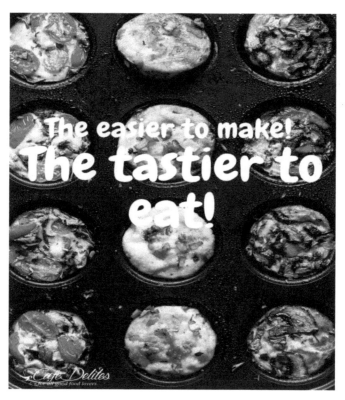

If you are in hurry, you can cook in extremely simple way by just beating eggs with salt and pepper and some onions. Then pouring the mixture into the pan and here is your dish ready. But if you have a little more time and you want to enjoy the meal, then follow the recipe and add your desired fillings to make the taste matchless.

This dish is not limited to just breakfast table, this can be included in picnic menu and you can also serve it to children as snack. Here is the formula to cook it!

Nutrition:

82 kcal | 1g carbs | 6g proteins | 5g fats

Ingredients:

- Eggs – 12
- Finely chopped spring onions – 2
- Cheddar cheese – ½ cup
- Red or green pesto
- Salt and pepper
- Dairy-free coconut milk (optional)

These are the basic ingredients. You can add some more to give it a better taste and a better look. You can use potatoes as well to make it a little heavier. Adding spinach, mint leaves, sun dried tomatoes will add beauty into it!

Instructions:

- Pre-heat the oven to 175° C or 350°F
- Take a muffin tin with insert able muffin cups. Grease it with butter to make it non sticky.

- Add the chopped spring onions (scallions) in the bottom of the tin.
- Whisk eggs with pesto, salt and pepper and make a mixture.
- Add cheese into the mixture and stir.
- Now add this mixture on top of the scallions in the tin.
- Bake it for 15 to 20 minutes and the cheesy keto egg muffins are ready!

Note:

- **Make sure to not heat the oven too much, otherwise the muffins will collapse. Let the muffins cool in the tin after taking it out from the oven, otherwise again your muffins will collapse.**
- **Use the non-sticky pans to avoid muffins sticking.**

Time saving hack: Cook the egg muffins by following above procedure. Then, place the tin into the freezer and freeze the muffins for future use. Next morning, you will just need to take a muffin out, heat it and eat it!

2- <u>Keto pancakes:</u>

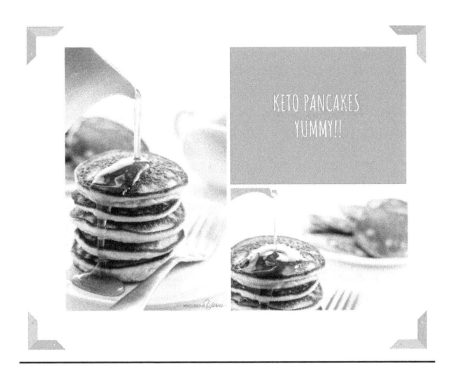

So easy, so fluffy and delicious. Low in carbs and high in fats and proteins. Best match for your breakfast table. There's nothing like a big stack of pancakes for breakfast— they're a classic breakfast staple! Just because you're on the Keto diet doesn't mean you have to miss out on the joys of flapjacks. This recipe is super easy and will definitely satisfy your craving.

Most of the people before following ketogenic diet think that the diet will contain boring medicine type foods. But no! It is not like you think, you can have almost every kind of meal you love but in a different way and with different ingredients.

There are other recipes for keto pancakes as well but they mainly involve two ingredients: Cream cheese and eggs. They also taste very good but you might not want something too eggy. In the recipe below, you will add almond flour and some other ingredients that will make your dish more caky and tasty.

Over light, fluffy pancakes but hate all the carbs? Let's make a keto pancakes recipe that is keto friendly. These almond flour pancakes take breakfast to the next level: low carb, gluten-free, and over-the-top tasty. These will be the best keto pancakes you will ever try.

The fluffier the better! This is the first thought that comes in your mind when you think of pancakes. Let's learn how to cook a fluffy pancake that is low carb and ketogenic in nature as well.

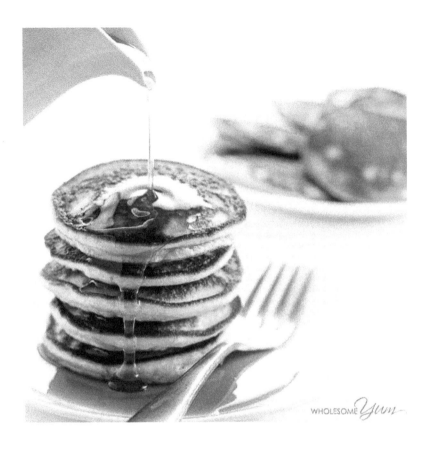

WHOLESOME *Yum*

When it comes to toppings, you have a lot of options. Traditionally if you are following ketogenic diet then you cannot use typical pancake toppings. Yet there are some ideas that you may like to consider. Toasted unsweetened coconut, a drizzle of melted unsweetened peanut butter, a handful of berries and a sprinkle of bacon, you can add some keto chocolate *chips as well. Oh! So yummy!!*

Nutrition:

391 kcal | 33g fats | 7.8g carbs | 14.9g proteins

Ingredients:

- Finely ground almond floor – 1 cup
- Coconut floor – ¼ cup
- Sweetener of your choice – 2-3 tsp
- Baking powder (Gluten-free) – 1 tsp
- Eggs – 5
- Almond milk (unsweetened) – 1/3 cup
- Any neutral tasting oil (e.g. Avocado oil etc.) – ¼ cup
- Vanilla extract (optional) – 1 ½ tsp
- Sea salt (optional) – ¼ tsp

As variation, you can add pepper as well. This would give it a little Italian taste. But it is not recommended most of the times.

Instructions

- Whisk all the ingredients in a bowl and prepare a smooth batter. Make sure the batter is not too thick.
- If the batter is too thick, add a little milk into it.
- Heat a pan over a stove with low to medium flame and preheat the oil.
- Drop the batter on the pan and make it in the form of circle.
- Cover and cook for 1-2 minutes. When bubbles form, flip and cook the other side for 1- 2 minutes until it becomes brown.
- Repeat the same process for remaining batter.

<u>Note:</u> If the batter is too thick, add a little milk into it. But not too much milk otherwise the cake will be wet.

<u>Time saving hack:</u> Cook the pancake and freeze it for the future use. Next morning, you will just need to take out the pancake from freezer, heat it and eat it!

3- <u>Ketogenic low carb cheese cake</u>

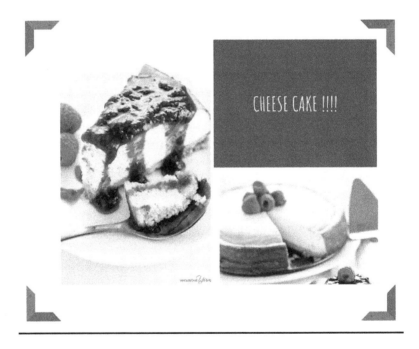

If you're looking for easy low carb keto cheesecake recipe you've come to the right place! A yummy cheese cake that is low carb, sugar free and gluten free. Sounds great, all in one package. This cheesecake is so rich, so smooth, and oh-so-creamy! It's a keto friendly shortbread cookie crust that'll have you forgetting about graham crackers in no time. This is an easy, tasty, budget friendly and time saving recipe.

It is really hard to find the difference between the normal cheese cake and the keto cheese cake. The only difference between the two is sweetener and the cake crust. The normal cheese cake recipes use a crust that is carb rich. In this recipe, the crust is made up of almond floor, butter and egg that makes it keto friendly. Moreover, the normal cake recipes include the use of sugar that is again high carb. In this recipe, sweetener is used instead of sugar to make it a keto meal.

In my opinion, cheesecake should be pure and decadent with only the essential ingredients...cream cheese, sweetener, eggs, vanilla, and sour cream.

Some of you might consider crust the most important thing of a keto cheese cake. The crust is delicious but not the most important. You can even make this recipe without the crust. In case you plan to cook a crust-less cake, you will need to grease the pan and line the bottom of pan with parchment paper.

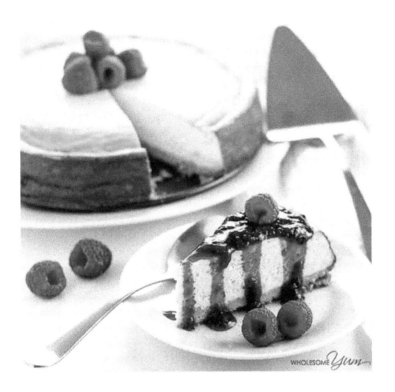

One more important thing that you must take care of is that all of the ingredients you are using must be at room temperature. The eggs cream and cheese must not be refrigerated.

There are some other tips that you may like to consider while making a keto cheese cake:

- ➤ For a smooth batter, use a powdered sweetener and not a liquid one.
- ➤ While beating the cream, add sweetener little by little. Make sure to beat the cream at slow seed.

➤ Beat the eggs one by one, then at last beat the sour cream and vanilla and mix well.

You can skip or add ingredients according to your choice.

So, what are you waiting for, boost up your keto diet with this yummy and fun recipe.

Nutrition:

600 kcal | 7g carbs | 14g proteins | 54g fats

Ingredients:

- Almond flour – 2 cups
- Butter – 1/3 cup
- Sweetener of your choice (erythritol etc.) – 1 ¼ tsp.
- Vanilla extract – 1 tsp.
- Cream cheese – 32 oz. (60 tsp.)
- Eggs – 3
- Lemon juice – 1 tsp.

These are the basic ingredients to make a yummy ketogenic cheese cake. You can add variations to satisfy your taste buds. You can use coconut flour. You can put different toppings once the cake is ready. Use raspberry sauce as topping to give your cake an excellent taste.

Instructions:

- Preheat the oven to 350°F or 177°C. Do not heat more than this otherwise cake will collapse.
- Grease the pan or line the bottom of pan with parchment paper so that the cake may not stick with the pan.

- To make the cake crust, mix the almond flour, vanilla extract, sweetener and melted butter in a bowl and stir it well and make dough.
- Press the dough on the bottom of the pan and bake it for 10-13 minutes.
- When the cake becomes barely golden, take it out and let it cool for about 10-15 minutes.
- Now take the cream cheese in a bowl and beat it with powdered sweetener until it becomes fluffy. Now add eggs one by one. Then add vanilla extract and lemon juice.
- Pour the cheese mixture over the cake crust in the pan. Smooth the top with a spatula.
- Bake for about 40-55 minutes until the center is almost set but still jiggle.
- Now remove the pan from the oven and let it cool to room temperature. Then refrigerate for at least 4 hours until completely set.
- Serve with fresh sauce if desired.

Note:

- *Do not beat the cheese mixture at fast speed otherwise the bubbles will form in the batter and it will ruin your cake. Make sure to beat it at slow or medium speed.*
- *Do not remove cake from the pan until chilled.*
- *Prepare the cake at night and then put in the freezer. Enjoy the cake at breakfast.*

4- Special ketogenic hot chocolate:

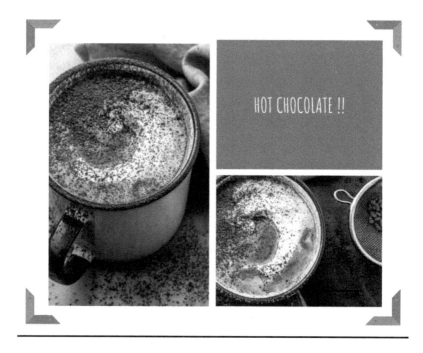

This Keto-Friendly Sugar-Free Hot Chocolate Recipe makes creamy, rich hot chocolate with ingredients you probably already have on hand. This quick and easy hot chocolate can be part of a low-carb, keto, diabetic, gluten-free, grain-free, Atkins or Banting diet. There is even a dairy-free option!

On a cold winter day, what can beat a great cup of keto hot chocolate? What is the secret behind making this delicious hot chocolate keto friendly? It's simple, the use of chocolate extract that also heightens the flavor as well!

Loaded with chocolate flavor, this recipe has got no match. Instead of sugar, sweetener is used to make it low carb. If you want to make it dairy-free, you will need to add thick dairy-free coconut milk instead of normal milk. This will also add coconut flavor that will please your heart as well.

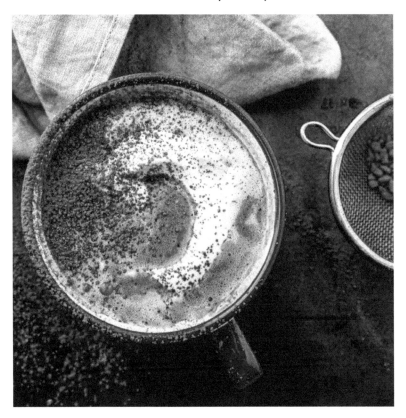

Another option to replace milk is to use heavy cream. This replacement will not only make it keto friendly but will also enhance the taste.

You can add almond butter and cocoa as extras. You can also sprinkle cocoa powder as topping when the hot chocolate is ready.

The best thing about ketogenic diet is that you can enjoy almost all meals you love but with a little variation. Mostly you need to replace sugar with some sugar free sweetener and to avoid dairy content. Sometimes, the ketogenic meal is richer in content and taste than the normal routine meals. This is a kind of diet that will not let you feel boring.

This recipe is quick and easy and it might become your favorite winter companion. A creamy hot chocolate that is unbeatable in taste and also ketogenic in nature. Yes! We are going to make something very yummy!

Nutrition:

193 kcal | 18g fats | 2g proteins | 4g carbs

Ingredients:

- Chopped chocolate chips (Sugar free) – 6 oz.
- Unsweetened almond mil – ½ cup
- Heavy cream – ½ cup
- Any sweetener of your choice – 1 tsp.
- Vanilla extract ½ tsp.

Variations are possible. You can give an almond or peanut finishing (topping) once the drink is ready. You can also use unsweetened normal milk instead of almond milk. Coconut milk is also an option. Variations depend on your taste buds!

Instructions:

- Take almond milk, cream and sweetener in a saucepan and put over a medium flame.
- When it simmers gently, remove it from heat.
- Now add vanilla extract and chocolate and stir it constantly until melted.
- Pour into cup and enjoy!

<u>Note</u>: *Do not let the milk become much thicker otherwise you will face problem during mixing the chocolate.*

<u>Tasty variation</u>:

- Once the hot chocolate is ready, pour almonds and peanuts to give it a better taste and look.
- Top the keto hot chocolate with whipped cream and a light dusting of cocoa powder.

5- <u>Ketogenic mushroom omelet</u>

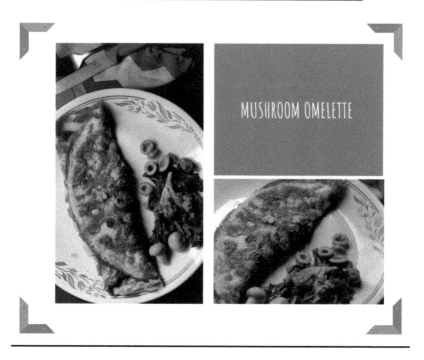

Breakfast has a great value in your keto diet plan. Eggs are a staple on the keto diet. This omelet is a nice breakfast but also would be good for lunch or dinner.

Omelets are always a great meal to make on the keto diet. Omelets are easy to whip up, full of good fats, filling, and taste so great! I love coming back to this recipe for an easy weeknight dinner when that breakfast for dinner craving hits, too!

The omelet is low carb and has a healthy amount of fats and protein. If you are looking for a quick and easy way to start your day then it is the right recipe for you. Yummy!! , It is a mouthwatering recipe. Not just yummy, it is ketogenic super healthy recipe. It is a type of recipe that you will continue even after your keto diet plan is completed. This recipe occupies a place in the long term memory and is very hard to forget.

Mushrooms are an interesting ingredient. When they are added into any dish, the increase the richness, taste and look by 100%. The onions form a perfect pair with mushrooms. The mushrooms give a smooth meaty bite while the onions will give a crunch.

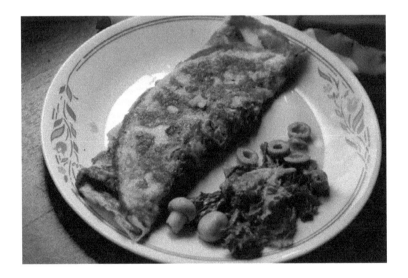

The addition of cheddar cheese enhances the taste as well. It gives a cheesy and creamy taste and makes the dressing beautifully pleasant.

If you give a little more time to do topping, then you are going to do a magic. Using mint leaves, red chili sauce as topping will add in taste. You can just sprinkle a little powdered black pepper and then feel the fragrance!

Fresh Mushrooms make a delicious appearance in the recipe. Very easy to make and is very less time consuming. You don't need to be a superman to make the dish, even if you've never cooked before; it is the suitable recipe for you to kick starts your cooking practice. Just take a pan and put it over stove and jump into the battle field of cooking.

Nutrition:

529 kcal | 6g carbs | 45g fats | 26g proteins

Ingredients:

- Sliced large mushrooms – 4
- Eggs – 3
- Butter for frying – 1 oz.
- Cheddar cheese – 4 tsp.
- Salt and pepper

These are the basic ingredients to make the dish. Variations are possible according to your wish. You can add green or red pesto as well. Adding mint is also an option.

Instructions:

- Take a bowl and crack the eggs into it. Add a pinch of salt and pepper and whisk it with a fork until smooth and frothy.

- Take the frying pan, put it on the flame and pour butter into it. Melt the butter over medium heat.
- Add the mushrooms and onions into the pan and heat until they become brownish.
- Now add the egg mixture into the pan over the mushroom and onions.
- When the omelet begins to cook and get firm, sprinkle cheese over the egg.
- Using a spatula, ease around the edges and fold it over in half. When it turns golden brownish in color, remove the pan from the flame and slide the omelet onto the plate.
- Sprinkle mint leaves over the omelet if you wish.
- The dish is ready, serve it to yourself and enjoy the dish.

Note:

- *Do not heat the pan too much over flame.*
- *Keep the flame low to medium otherwise the omelet will burn.*

Extras: You can add mint leaves as an extra. This will enhance the taste very much. Or you can sprinkle black pepper to give it a beautiful fragrance.

6- <u>Special ketogenic iced coffee</u>

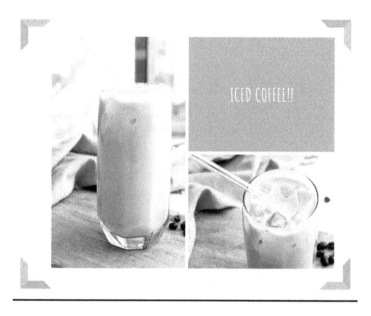

Coffee is an ultimate breakfast companion for most of the people. Morning seems to be ceased if there is no coffee on the table. Coffee is the real beauty of breakfast table. Most of the professional people skip coffee in the breakfast but as soon as they reach office or work place. The first thing that they need to kick start the work is a cup of coffee. But as a ketogenic diet follower, you cannot rely on outdoor coffee as it can contain high carb content that will ruin your keto diet plan. So you would surely need to spend a little time for your tummy!

This coffee not only boost energy levels but also promotes ketosis in body and as a result fat starts burning. It depends on you whether you want to have a hot coffee or a cold one, taste in both cases has got no match.

If you want to promote more ketosis, you can add coconut oil with your black coffee before icing it. You can also mix sugar-free flavorings such as vanilla extract or cinnamon extract. You may also like to use MCT oil powder to flavor your coffee.

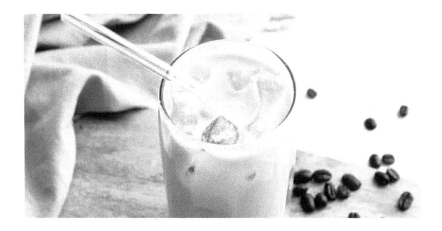

Again it is not a difficult or time consuming recipe. You have to go to office, No problem! This recipe doesn't demand a lot of time. So, keep your sleeves up and let's make a cup of iced coffee that is low in carbs and is a ketosis agent as well!

But yes! There remains a challenge to make your coffee keto. So there are two ways to do so. You can buy a 'keto coffee' from the store nearby or you can make it at home by using different keto ingredients. If you've got a keto coffee from store, than the procedure to make it similar to making normal coffee. But in other case, you need to follow the following recipe!

Nutrition:

160 kcal | 16g fats | 1.5g carbs | 1.6g protein

Ingredients:

- Heavy cream – 3 tsp.
- Vanilla extract – ½ tsp.
- Ice cubes – as required
- Liquid stevia – 5 drops
- Coffee – 1 cup

Instructions:

- First of all prepare the coffee in normal way as you make it and let it cool to room temperature.
- Now add ice cubes in it.
- Add heavy cream, stevia and vanilla extract into the coffee.
- Mix it with a spoon and enjoy the tasty, yummy, ketogenic coffee.

Note:

- *If you want to make it quick and cannot wait to let it cool , you can put it in refrigerator for a while. Do not add ice cubes into the hot coffee otherwise your coffee would start looking like water.*
- *You can skip vanilla extract if you want. Moreover, you can skip cream as well if black coffee is fine for you.*

Time saving hack: Make a jug of coffee and put it in the refrigerator. Next morning, you will just need to pour the coffee into the cup and mix other ingredients and enjoy the coffee within 60 seconds!

7- <u>Mushroom frittata with goat cheese</u>

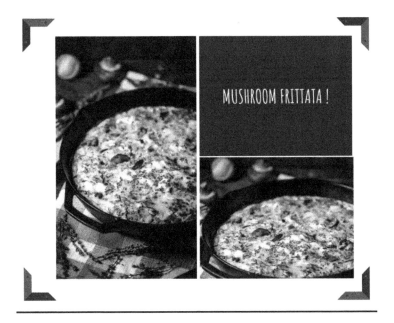

Elevate your breakfast or brunch with this fancy yet approachable Mushroom Goat Cheese Frittata! This recipe is ready in just over 30 minutes and even works well for meal prep.

The beauty of ketogenic diet is that it is not only for non-veg people but also for the vegetarians as well. Mushroom frittata is one of the best ketogenic recipes for vegetarian people. Alike other recipe, again this is an easy to make, time saving, delicious and healthy recipe.

This mushroom frittata with goat's cheese makes an economically and medically moderate breakfast. It's great as a breakfast, for a picnic and sometimes for a beautiful night dinner.

A frittata is a versatile egg dish that can be tweaked and tailored to your tastes. You may like to consider bacon cheddar version of frittata as well. The earthiness of the mushrooms pair beautifully with tangy goat cheese, and a handful of fresh herbs ties it all together.

It's not just the taste; its look will make you love it. You may forget its taste after some years but still you would remember its look. Oh! It looks like a pizza, a tasty mushroom pizza. Cheesy, creamy and juicy. Everything a human's tongue needs just in one plate. It's so yummy and easy to make, you can serve it to your tummy if you are alone. If you have children, make this for them as a healthy snack and they would love such a snack. If you are married, serve it to your husband and he would just eat his fingers up.

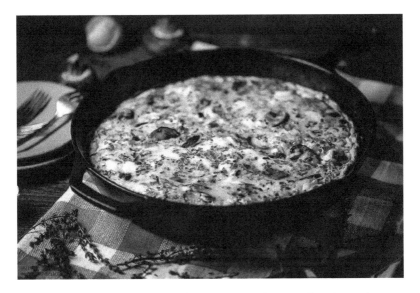

This is an Italian recipe with an eggy richness that is truly enjoyable. It only takes about 30 minutes to be ready which makes it convenient meal! Let's take a step ahead and occupy the kitchen!

Nutrition:

207 kcal | 7g carbs | 12g protein | 15g fats

Ingredients:

- Eggs – 8
- Unsweetened milk (dairy-free) – ¼ cup
- Goat cheese – 3 ounces
- Cooking oil – 2 tsp.
- Diced onion – ½ piece
- Mushrooms – 6 ounces
- Baby spinach chopped – 3 ounces
- Salt and pepper

These are the basic ingredients but you can add variations of your choice as well. I recommend adding a little mint and pepper sausage as topping.

Instructions:

- Preheat the oven to 425° F. Grease the pan (skillet) with 2 spoons of cooking oil.
- Add the diced onion into the pan for about two minutes before adding the sliced mushrooms.
- Cook the mushrooms and onions for 6-8 minutes until they release their moisture and have begun to brown.
- Add the baby spinach to the skillet and stir it with the mushrooms.
- When spinach is wilted, remove the vegetables from skillet and grease it with butter or oil.
- Now again add the vegetables into the skillet and spread them evenly over it.
- Take a bowl and beat the eggs with milk, salt and pepper. Pour the egg mixture over the vegetables in the skillet.
- Place the skillet back on the burner. Cook for about 5 minutes over the stove until the bottom and edges begin to set and have just begun to firm up then add the pieces of goat cheese over the top of the frittata.
- Put the skillet into the hot oven and bake for 8- 10 minutes until the eggs have set.
- And here is the ready to eat Ketogenic mushroom frittata with goat cheese. Taste it and forget the boring world!

Note: To make this dish with a better taste, you will need both the stove burner and the oven.

<u>Tips:</u> This dish is not limited to just breakfast table. You can take it with you for a picnic. You just need to cut triangular pieces and pack them in plastic sheet. This frittata is long lasting and doesn't become loose like sandwich.

If you are not vegetarian and you want to enjoy the dish as well, you can add BBQ chicken or beef pieces to give it a shape and taste of a BBQ pizza

8- <u>Ketogenic veggie scrambled eggs</u>

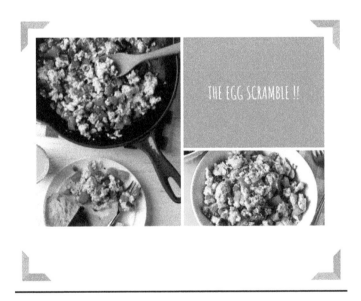

You can make up a warm, satisfying meal on beautiful winter mornings just like this veggie scrambled eggs that is

low carb breakfast. Yes, there are a lot time saving breakfasts like you just take freezer breakfast sandwiches etc. , heat them and have a breakfast. But nothing can be better than a fresh cooked breakfast that you cook with your own hands and along with the ingredients you add a bit of love and this love gives an unbeatable flavor to your breakfast.

Scrambled eggs with sautéed mushrooms and peppers are topped with Parmesan cheese and fresh cut green onions. Delicious, fast, easy, and oh-so keto.

 If you are a vegetarian, it will be a challenging task for you to decide your meal for breakfast. Yes! Pancakes or cheese cakes might be a good option but you cannot stick to a single meal every morning as your tongue has rights to taste different things as well. Sometimes, your tongue may be satisfied after eating sweet breakfast including keto cakes but other times it will need a little salty and chili flavor to be satisfied. So, don't fight against your tongue, keep reading and prepare a recipe that is really worthy of your tongue!

You need to be a little creative to cook this dish. Just a few seasonings and you can whip up a tasty. Vegan version of scrambled eggs in matter of minutes!

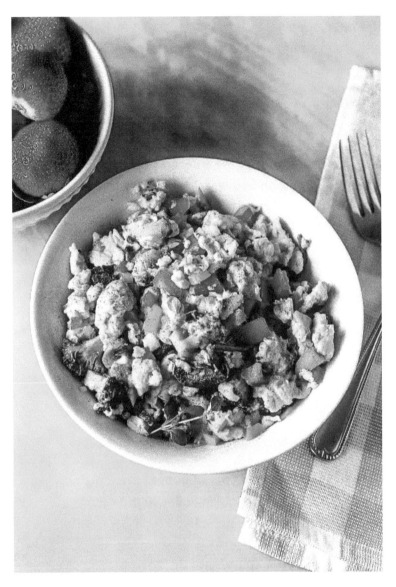

The base of this recipe uses firm tofu seasoned with nutritional yeast for a cheesy flavor. You can also add a bit of turmeric to add a bit more flavor and a beautiful color. Addition of diced onion, spinach and a bit of cheddar cheese will make it delicious.

It is not just delicious but is also easy to make. You just put veggies in a pan; add whisked eggs and everything is cooked up. But for sure your creativity will add a lot of flavoring to it.

For saving your time, you can have your veggies already cut and diced and freeze. In this case you will just need to take the veggies out of the freezer, put them into the pan, when they heat up, add eggs and you have your scrambled eggs ready. It is a good option for those who are job doers and do not have much time to cut the veggies in the morning. But for those who have time, freshly cut veggies are always recommended.

Nutrition:

This beautifully tasty diet is keto friendly. The nutrition content in the diet is as follows:

211.4g calories | 17.56g fats | 6.88g carbs | 10.09g proteins.

Ingredients:

- Firm tofu package – 14 ounce
- Avocado oil or cooking oil – 3tsp
- Diced yellow onion – 2tsp
- Yeast – 1 ½ tsp
- Garlic powder – ½ tsp
- Turmeric and salt – ½ tsp
- Vegan cheddar cheese – 3 ounce
- Tomatoes - 3
- Baby spinach – 1 cup

Instructions:

- Take block of tofu and put it on few layers of water. Squeeze a little to remove some water out of it and set it aside.
- Heat the cooking oil in a pan over a stove and add chopped onions into it until soft.
- Now place the tofu block into the pan and crumble it using a fork or masher until it is evenly mashed like scrambled eggs.
- Drizzle with the rest of the oil and sprinkle with the dry seasoning then gently stir to coat.
- Cook the scramble over low to medium flame until most of the liquid is evaporated.
- Keep stirring and folding the scramble so that it may not stick with the pan.
- Now add baby spinach, tomatoes and cheese into the pan and cook the scramble for a minute or until the spinach wilts and the cheese are melted.
- Serve it hot! And store the leftover in the refrigerator for future use.
- This recipe will give you 5 servings of ketogenic veggie scrambled eggs.

Note:

- *Stir and fold continuously otherwise the scramble will stick to the pan.*
- *Keep the flame low to medium otherwise the scramble may get burnt*

- *Squeeze the tofu block to release some water before cooking otherwise it will take more time to cook.*

9- Delicious Ketogenic taco omelet

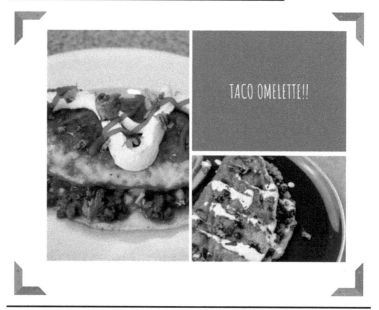

You have come to the right place if you were looking for a quick and hearty keto meal that keeps you satiated for a long time and its taste would keep you memorizing it again and again. A very good way to start you keto day, perfect for breakfast.

This is a Mexican recipe that will burst taste into your heart. If you are a fan of cheese shell tacos then this cheesy taco omelet is going to change the way you think about taste of something. It is a more than perfect combination of yummy eggs, cheese and Mexican flavors. This meal is not limited to just breakfast table, you can serve it on the lunch or dinner table as well. This Mexican inspired cheesy omelet would be perfect as a snack as well during any time of the day.

The base of omelet contains egg and cheese combination and that works perfectly. The cheese provides some crunch when it is cooked and the eggs keep the cheese from setting too hard.

As for taco, you will have to be a little careful while buying taco from market as most of the companies have added sugar to tacos that is not keto friendly. So you would have to be careful and must buy sugar free tacos.

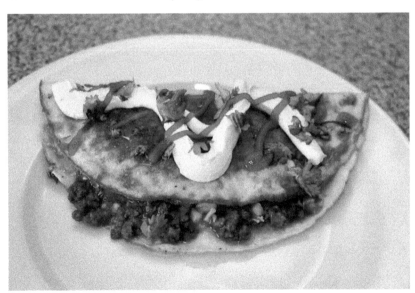

Once you have mastered the omelet base, then you have a whole universe of fillings and you can chose what satisfies your taste buds. Some great options for fillings are:

- ❖ Ham, mushroom and onion
- ❖ Spinach and feta
- ❖ Pimento Cheese
- ❖ Shredded beef or chicken

These fillings are mostly included as Mexican fillings. If these are not what you like, you can add something else with your creative mind. This recipe is all about you creativity and imagination. Some other add ons that you may get interested in are:

- ❖ Avocado
- ❖ Sour cream, oh yummy!
- ❖ Hot sauce
- ❖ Chilies
- ❖ Spring onions
- ❖ Mint leaves

As said before, there is whole universe of ingredients that you can add into this recipe. You just need to spark your creativity and imagination and the whole universe will be yours.

Nutrition:

8g carbs, 63g fat, 44g protein, 790 kcal

Ingredients:

Now let us talk about the basic ingredients to prepare the recipe.

- Ground beef (beef mince) – 100 g
- Taco seasoning – ½ tsp
- Eggs – 2
- Cheddar cheese (Grated) – 85 g
- Salt and pepper – as required

Optional ingredients:

- Sour cream
- Avocado
- Hot sauce

Instructions:

- Put a pan over a stove and heat the ground beef in the pan until meat is browned and shows goldish color.
- Add the taco seasoning and cook for a while until the beef is completely cooked. Now set the beef aside.
- Take a bowl and whisk eggs with salt and pepper.
- Now pour grated cheese into the bottom of the pan, spread evenly and cook until the cheese is bubbling.
- Now pour the egg mixture over the cheese and cook on low flame for 2-4 minutes.
- When the egg mixture is set, pour the beef mixture over the half omelet and cook for further 2 minutes.
- Carefully fold the cheese and egg mixture side of the omelet over the top of beef mixture side of the omelet and cook for 2 minutes more.

- When the omelet is set, transfer it to a plate and top it with your desired combination of toping and enjoy the meal.

Note:

Do not stir when you add eggs over the cheese.

Keep the flame low to medium, otherwise cheese base may get burnt from outside.

10-   <u>Basil and butter scramble with eggs.</u>

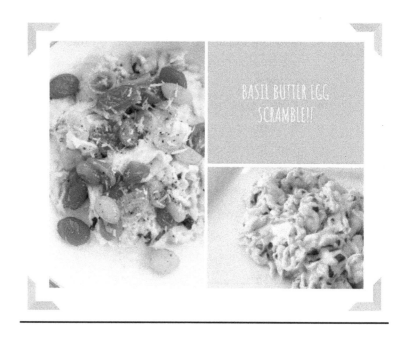

A clever and elegantly simple version of a keto scrambled eggs with cream. Cheese, herbs and juicy butter. What else you need to kick start your day if you have such a delicious breakfast. Creamy and cheesy, it's so filling, you'll be able to push back lunch.

If you are following specific diet then it is very important for you to have a delicious and filling breakfast that is low in carbs and is also healthier. Well the most common and classic option is using eggs as keto breakfast yet you may want to add some flavor into the eggs as well. Moreover, you cannot eat eggs daily because you will be fed up of eating a same thing again and again. You will definitely want to switch your routine.

This is a recipe that will add an amazing flavor to your boring classic eggs breakfast and will help you make your morning eggs exciting while keeping them easy to prepare.

You will notice one thing while preparing this recipe that it is full of fat with cream cheese and butter. And you already know that fat is an essential part of keto diet. Keto diet is in fact the intake of fats every day so that your body may forget about carbs and start consuming the fat as energy source. So all of the fats in this recipe not only add amazing flavor, making the eggs creamy and irresistible, but they also promote a healthy keto diet.

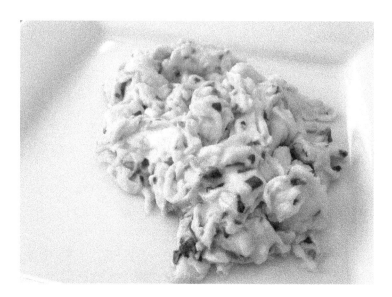

This recipe is not just offering fats so that your diet plan may get running in a boring way, rather its main offer is its taste! These eggs soaked in basil butter give a fresh taste.

Basil adds an unbeatable flavor to this recipe when you add fresh chopped basil into melted butter and cream cheese. It imparts its strong taste when the basil is blended with other ingredients. This basil butter combination is used as toping over the eggs and its look and taste both will make your mouth water.

With lots of great keto fats, an abundant amount of fresh flavors and a meal you can make in just a few minutes, this recipe is a sure win. Keep it in mind for an easy weekday breakfast and a way to make your classic egg dishes new again!

Nutrition:

359 calorie, 30g fat, 18g protein, 2g net carbs.

Ingredients:

- Eggs – 4
- Cream cheese – 2 tsp
- Shredded mozzarella cheese – ¼ cup
- Butter – 2 tsp
- Chopped fresh basil – 2 tsp
- Salt and ground black pepper – as required

Instructions:

- Take a small bowl and add one spoon of butter and cream cheese along with one table spoon of basil and microwave for about 20-30seconds until melt. Stir the mixture to combine fully and add mozzarella and set aside to cool slightly.
- Take another bowl and whisk eggs in it with salt and pepper. Then add the basil butter mixture into it and whisk well.
- Heat the butter in a pan over medium heat and pour the egg mixture into the pan and cook. Make sure to stir constantly to scramble eggs.
- When the eggs are cooked, transfer them to a plate and pour the remaining basil over it as topping and enjoy the meal!

Note:

- *Keep the flame low otherwise the egg mixture will burn*

- *Make sure to stir continuously otherwise the mixture will stick to the pan.*

Ketogenic lunch recipes

When you think of keto diet, you may regret when you will not be able to eat bread, bagels or baguettes, your favorite burgers and sandwiches etc. But when you have look on the things that you can eat during the diet plan, the keto feels much more achievable.

Ketogenic diet is a vast diet plan that contains a lot of recipes that are different according to the region you live in and also according to the taste buds of different people. The most beautiful thing about the diet is that it is not just for one group of people (non-veg) but is for the both groups. There are recipes that suits best the requirements of non-veg people and there are also a lot of recipes that suit best for the vegetarian people as well.

Following ketogenic lunch recipes are for both groups of people. With delicious non-veg recipes and unbeatably tasty veg recipes, the list is going to rock!

The list is made by taking in account the basic requirements for a diet to be called as ketogenic meal. Nutrient content is written with each recipe showing low carbs content. Mostly the recipes avoid use of the ingredients that contain high carb content and just those ingredients are included that are low in carbs and high in fats and proteins.

Get yourself pack up! We are going to dive into a whole ocean of Ketogenic lunch recipes.

Non-Vegetarian ketogenic recipes

A ketogenic diet with toppings of meat balls on one hand and shredded beef on the other hand. The most delicious combinations sometimes filled up with juicy and creamy cheese and sometimes with chilies that would take you to another world.

This list of recipes is for the non-veg people and mostly contains recipes where meat is used. Next list will contain meat-free recipes for the vegetarian people.

1- ketogenic paleo baked meatballs recipe

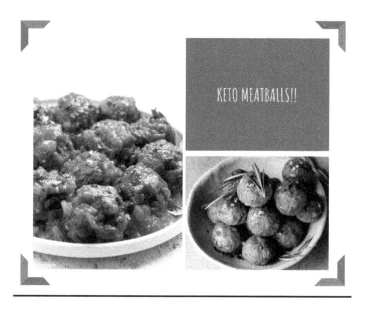

The meatballs make the perfect option for busy day routines as it doesn't take a lot of time to prepare this meal.

It's always been a great topic of debate between the cooks that whether the meatballs should be baked or pan fried. For the best flavor, it is mostly recommended to pan fry them. Pan frying meatballs produces superior caramelization and a flavorful outer crust, but the meatballs rarely retain their round shape. There is also a problem in pan frying and that the meatballs will not retain the round shape and they will look squarer than the balls.

In this recipe, baking and frying both are combined in order to give you the best tasty flavor as well as the best look that will please your eyes. In this combined approach, the meatballs are partially baked to get round shape and then these are finished over a frying pan to give them an unbeatable flavor.

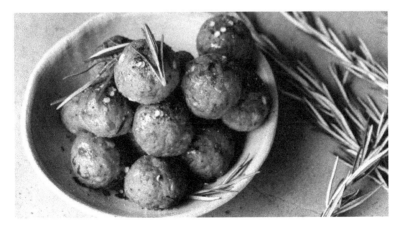

Meatballs and are not juicy? This is not the desired meal! If one is making meatballs, the first priority is to make them juicy. This recipe has a treatment for this problem as well. You will just need to use heavy cream to give your meatballs moisture and a little more fat. Mostly people use bread or bread crumbs to give moisture to meatballs but it is against the requirements of a ketogenic meal. Bread is a high carb ingredient and will ruin your keto diet plan in minutes. So, the best choice remains are to use heavy cream.

Nutrition:

38g fats | 1g carbs | 19g proteins are included per serving.

Ingredients:

- Ground beef – ½ pounds
- Grated parmesan cheese – ¼ cup
- Heavy cream – ¼ cup
- Egg – 1 large
- Minced fresh parsley – 2 tsp
- Finely grated onion – 1 tsp
- Garlic – 1 grated
- Salt and pepper – as required
- Optional sauce – Rao's Marinara sauce 2 cups

Instructions:

- Take a bowl and add ground beef into it by breaking into smaller chunks aiming for an even mix.

- Add the other ingredients into the beef and mix with the hand mixer until combined. Do not over mix.
- Now grease your hands with oil and roll 20 meat balls out of the beef. Make sure to roll the balls in equal weights for even cooking.

To bake the meat balls:

- Pre heat oven to 400°F . Put the meatballs into the foil lined baking sheet and place into the oven.
- Partially bake the meatballs for 10-15 minutes.

To fry the partially baked meatballs:

- Put a frying pan over medium flame of stove. If the pan is stainless, non-sticky, it will be a plus point. When pan is hot, pour in the oil (2 tsp) and let it heat for few seconds.
- Add partially baked meatballs into the pan one by one. Make sure to not crowd the pan too much otherwise the meatballs will be steamed and become tough.
- Cook the meatballs for about 1-1.5 minutes per side turning at least 4 times. Cook until the meat is set and the balls must look browned.
- Now heat the sauce in the pan a little bit to give it a nice flavor. For a fresh taste of sauce, pour the warm sauce over meatballs. Top them with parsley or some other toping that you like and serve with melted mozzarella cheese. Oh so yummy!!

Some tasty variations:

Variations depend on your imagination and creativity. However, you can sprinkle a pinch of black pepper over the hot ready meatballs; this will give them an exceptional taste. Make a mint leaves sauce and dip the meatballs into it to increase the taste up to a high level. Using heavy cream as a toping is also an option but is not recommended mostly. Red chili sauce will also give an exceptional look when placed along the meatballs over lunch table. You can add any other ingredient that according to your imagination fits best in the recipe.

Note:

Do not mix the beef and eggs mixture too much otherwise the meatballs will not stick together and will be spread in the pan.

Time saving hack:

Prepare the beef and eggs mixture, roll out meatballs and place in the freezer. Whenever you want to eat the dish, take meatballs out, bake and fry and enjoy!

2- <u>Low carb dairy-free butter chicken</u>

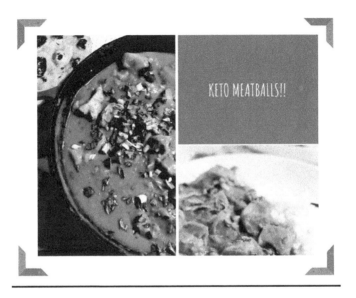

An Indian classic recipe that you will love more than anything. Slow cooker dairy-free butter chicken recipe made with coconut oil and coconut milk loaded with flavor.

You will love to know that the keto butter is one of the most beloved Indian dishes. It's a popular dish with chicken in a spiced tomato, butter and cream sauce or gravy.

The recipe below contains a little variation in the traditional butter chicken recipe. The variation is to skip the cream to make the dish 100% dairy-free. Traditionally, the chicken is marinated in yogurt mixture but instead of yogurt, you will be using coconut milk and skipping the marinating process completely. Chicken without marinating? Does it sound strange? Don't worry at all, the slow cooker ensures the meat has plenty of time to soak up all the flavors added to it?

Another variation is skipping the butter. You will be using coconut oil instead of butter to make the dish completely dairy free. This replacement doesn't affect the taste at all but it provides the same robust richness. If you cook of onion, garlic, and ginger before placing all the ingredients in the slow cooker, that will be a plus point as it enhances the taste and the fragrance.

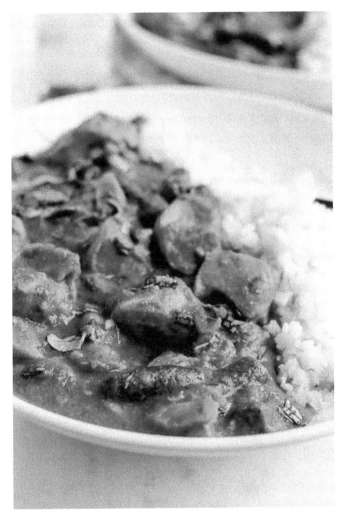

Remember, you don't need to limit yourself to classic traditional recipe. Let your creativity make this recipe tastier and tastier. You can add different variations such as vegetables, beans etc. You can also have cauliflower rice with heavy sprinkle of chopped cilantro and a squeeze of lime. In traditional recipes there is no use of beans or vegetables but if you use them, you will not be sent to the jail. So, feel free and let your imagination and creativity make magical tastes.

The best thing about Indian dishes is that they not only taste and look good, but they also smell a lot of good. Your kitchen will burst with a greatly enjoyable fragrance of all the ingredients you will use in recipe.

When we talk about Indian recipes, the first thing that comes in mind is that the dish would be extra spicy. It is true to some extent but not for this recipe. It is moderately spicy due to cayenne pepper but that much spice is bearable when it tastes like hell. Whereas, you can skip the pepper if you don't want much spice or add more if you want to make it spicier.

So, let's make a lightened version of an Indian classic recipe.

Nutrition:

304 calories, 18g fats, 9g carbs, 2g fiber, 28g protein

Ingredients:

- Coconut oil – 2 tsp
- Boneless chicken (Chopped chunks) – 2 lb
- Cinnamon (Grounded) – ½ tsp
- Cayenne (optional) – ½ tsp
- Chili powder – 1 tsp
- Garam masala – 1 tsp
- Turmeric (grounded) – 2 tsp
- Ginger (chopped) – 1 inch knob
- Garlic (minced) – 5 cloves

- Yellow onion (chopped) – 1
- Cumin – 1 tsp
- Salt – as required
- Coconut milk – 15 oz
- Tomato sauce – 15 oz
- Lemon juice – 2 tsp
- Green beans (optional) – 2 cups
- Cilantro (chopped) – ¼ cup
- 1 cinnamon stick

Instructions:

- Add oil to a large skillet or saucepan and cook onion and garlic until soft and fragrant, about 5 minutes.
- Add fresh ginger, turmeric, garam masala, cumin, chili powder, salt, pepper, cinnamon and cayenne and toss to combine. Cook for another 1-2 minutes. (This step can be done in the base of your slow cooker if it allows.)
- Transfer onion and garlic mixture into your slow cooker. Add chicken, coconut milk, tomato sauce, lemon juice and cinnamon stick to the slow cooker as well. Cover and cook on high for 3 hours or low for 6 hours. Add green beans when there's about 1 hour left in the cooking process.
- Serve over cauliflower rice (optional) with fresh cilantro and a wedge of lemon for squeezing.

Note:

- It is a slow cooker recipe; you will need to spend time over it. Don't cook it over high flame; otherwise it will be of no use.
- Cook the onion, ginger, garlic paste a little before you add other ingredients.

3- Ketogenic fat-head pizza

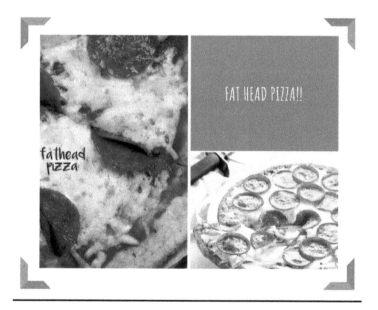

Best pizza ever! All flavors that you love, layered on top of a crunchy and cheesy keto crust. Oh! That's yummy!! Fat head pizza is the ultimate keto pizza. Its recipe makes it ketogenic when crust is made with coconut flour or almond flour that is low carb ingredient.

This recipe starts with the shredded mozzarella cheese and a little cream cheese. Then the addition of eggs and almond flour give it a heroic and tasty look. If you add a little bit of Italian seasoning it will boost the flavor but it is an optional thing to do.

Those who have tried the keto fathead pizza may know that there is a lot similar between the taste of a normal pizza and a keto fat head pizza. For sure, if you have to pizzas in front of you, one is normal pizza and other is keto pizza and you have to identify which one is keto it will become really difficult for you to do so. The main difference is the difference of pizza dough. The normal pizza dough is made up of wheat while fathead pizza dough is made up of some low carb flour mixed with cream cheese, eggs and mozzarella.

The thing that makes this recipe ketogenic is that it is gluten-free and sugar free. There's a reason fathead pizza crust is such a staple for a keto diet plan. Its super easy to make, and the best part is that the texture is very close to real pizza!

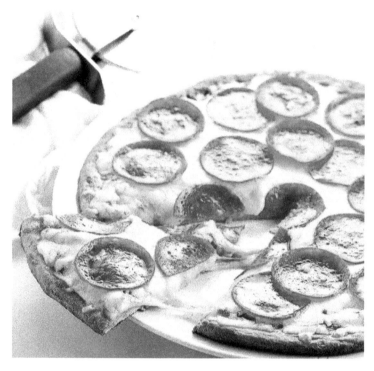

This Fathead pizza recipe tastes pretty much like regular pizza! And the texture is spot-on, which is one of the most challenging things to get right with low carb dough.

When it comes to toppings, this not a difficult job as most of the pizza toppings are naturally low carb including meat, mushrooms and vegetables. So you have a choice, if you are non-veg, you can add meat as topping. If you are vegetarian, you have a whole galaxy of vegetable to use as topping.

Why we call it 'fathead' pizza?

So, it's an interesting story. The recipe has been gone viral since 2013 when Tom Naughton posted it for the first time. The name comes from the blog Tom Naughton started while making the movie Fat Head, a comedy documentary about food and health.

Nutrition:

235 calories | 19g fats | 4g carbs | 18g protein

Ingredients for crust:

- Shredded mozzarella cheese – 1 ½ cup
- Cream cheese – 2 tsp
- Vinegar – 1tsp
- Almond flour – ¾ cups
- 1 egg
- Salt – as required
- Oil to grease your hands

Ingredients for topping:

- Fresh Italian sausage – 8 oz
- Butter – 1tsp
- Unsweetened tomato sauce – ½ cup
- Shredded mozzarella cheese – 1 ½ cups

Instructions:

- Put a non-sticky pan over a medium flame and heat mozzarella and cream cheese in it. Stir and melt them together. Then add other ingredients and well with hand mixer.
- Grease your hands with oil and put the dough on parchment paper evenly. Flatten the dough evenly.
- Pre-heat the oven to 200°C/400°F

- Remove the parchment sheet, prick the crust with a fork and bake in the oven for 10-15 minutes until it becomes golden brown.
- While the crust is baking, cook the sausage meat in olive oil or butter a little bit.
- Take the baked crust out, spread a thin layer of tomato sauce on the crust. Top the pizza with meat and a lot of cheese. Bake again for 10-15 minutes until the cheese melts.
- Sprinkle olives and mint leaves and enjoy your meal!

Time saving hack:

Make extra crusts and store them for 2-3 days in the fridge or in the freezer for up to 2 months. The pizza reheats great in the microwave so if you get left-overs, and you probably will because this is very rich, enjoy them in the next day's lunch box.

4-Keto Tortilla Española

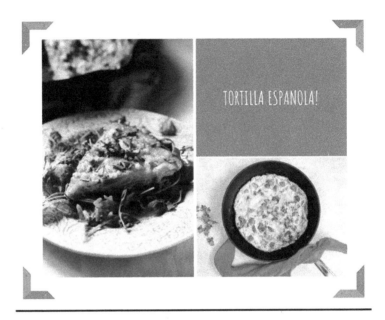

TORTILLA ESPANOLA!

So, this yummy recipe basically belongs to Spanish origin. What we have done is that we took recipe of a Spanish omelet and converted it into the ketogenic diet recipe. Fact is, this keto tortilla Española manages to taste like the real thing. Pretty amazing really. Layer after layer of onions and potatoes cooked in extra virgin olive oil into smooth perfection. Beauty of this meal is that its scope is not limited to lunch table only, you can cook it in the morning for breakfast, and you can enjoy it at dinner or on picnic as well.

And yes, like most of the keto recipes, it is also not a difficult one to make. You just need to slice your radishes and onions and cook them slowly in olive oil until they become smooth like silk.

You've to make choice about the cooking method. If you have a very good non sticky pan then you can make it as double turn tortilla method. Otherwise it's recommended that you simply cook it frittata style.

Again, the question of toppings! Like all other keto recipes this one also puts the question of toppings over your imagination and creativity. Traditional tortilla Española is made with just potatoes, onions and eggs garnished with fresh parsley and served up with spinach or arugula. But as always said, you don't need to stick to traditions always. You can add some other combination of toppings as well. Light sprinkle of feta cheese prior to baking will be a wonderful option.

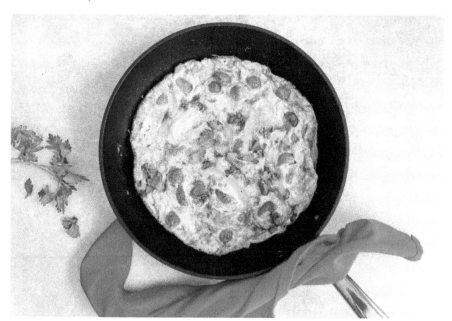

Now we come to the choice of vegetables. The choice again rests with your taste buds. Yet some options should be discussed as well. Spinach, asparagus and mushrooms are recommended if you are confused in the matter of choosing vegetables. To give the recipe more flavor and crunch, you can add cooked chopped bacon as well. You may like to add ham pieces to add a different texture and taste.

Nutrition:

139kcal | 2.35g carbs | 6.95g proteins | 8.56g fat

Ingredients:

- Mushrooms (sliced) – 1 cup
- Baby spinach – 2 cups
- 1 yellow onion
- 7 eggs
- Olive oil – 4 tsp
- Smoked paprika – ½ tsp
- Grated jack cheese – ½ cup
- Spears asparagus – 3 inch
- Strips bacon – 3 inch
- Red pepper – as required

Instructions:

- Take a non-sticky pan, better if you have a double sided pan. Heat olive oil in it over a medium flame. Take another pan and add 1tsp olive oil in it and put it over low flame on another burner.

- Add asparagus and mushrooms to the first pan and cook until set. Add spinach, pepper and chopped bacon, stir together then set aside off burner.
- Now take a bowl and beat eggs with vegetable mixture and cheese, stirring together so that eggs may not begin to scramble.
- Now put the whole mixture back into the first pan and cook over a medium flame until set.
- Drain out oil from the second pan and flip the first pan over the second pan.
- Cook until tortilla becomes slightly brown.
- Now transfer the tortilla into the plate and enjoy the meal!

Note:

A two sided pan is mostly available in homes nowadays. If you don't have one and are making the recipe in a skillet then be careful while flipping the tortilla.

5- Special ketogenic Lamb kofta kebabs

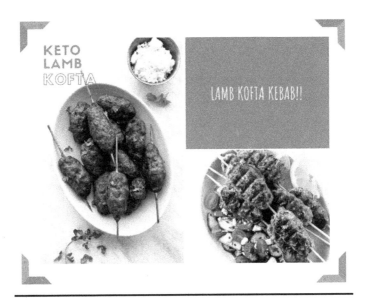

In all seriousness though, these low-carb koftas are super-fast and easy to make. The longest part of the whole dish is soaking your skewers in cold water so that they don't burn. If you add a cool keto friendly mint leaves sauce, it will add in deliciousness of the recipe.

The real beauty of this recipe is again that it is not difficult to cook. You need to get minced lamb meat and add few spices and other ingredients into it. Then make a yummy delicious sauce and enjoy the meal!

What is kofta?

Kofta is basically a word that belongs to eastern region. This is similar to meatballs or meatloaf. It is a mixture of minced meat formed into shape of a ball. Different versions of Kofta are made using different kinds of meat such as beef, chicken, lamb and a variety of spices.

Once you have the kofta kebabs ready, you can add a lot of variations to enhance the look and taste. Some of the best recommended variations are as follows.

Keto Naan bread – This pita-liked bread looks perfect if wrapped around your lamb kofta.

Serving with salads – When it comes to salads, there are options you have to choose. You can either make creamy cucumber salad as a side keto dish or Mediterranean salad with sun dried tomato. It depends upon your taste buds, you have to make a choice that best satisfies your tongue.

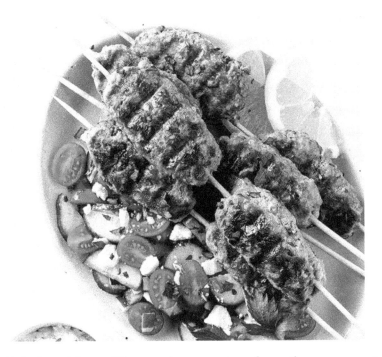

Kebabs with cauliflower rice – as clear from the name, put the kebabs on a plate full of cauliflower rice, oh! So yummy!

You can also make variety of sauces. Spicy sauces fit the best with the kebab but if you don't like much spices, you can have sauce of your own choice.

Another interesting variation is also possible for those who don't love lamb meat. What is beef for? You don't like lamb, leave it! Buy grounded (minced) beef instead and follow the same recipe and satisfy your tummy!

Kofta is really quite similar to meatballs or hamburger patties, so it's very simple to make. It can be served on skewers, which is fun but not necessary. And it can be grilled, pan-fried, or baked.

Nutrition:

437 calories | 27.4g fata | 1.8g carbs | 37.9g Protein

Ingredients:

- Ground lamb meat – 2 lb
- 8 bamboo skewers
- Grated onion – ¼ cup
- Minced garlic – 2 cloves
- Chopped fresh parsley – 1 tsp
- Cumin – 1 tsp
- Black pepper – ¼ tsp

Instructions:

- Soak the bamboo skewers in water for 30 minutes.
- Meanwhile, in a large bowl, stir together all ingredients except the lamb. Add the lamb and mix until just combined. Do not over-mix.
- Divide the meat into 16 sections. Mold each section of meat around a bamboo skewer, making it a few inches long and about 1 inch (2.5 cm) thick. You'll fit 2 sections of meat per skewer, about 1-2 inches apart.
- Preheat the grill to medium-high heat and oil the grates lightly. Place the skewers on the grill and cook for 3 minutes. Flip and cook for 3-5 more minutes, to desired level of doneness. Time on the second side will be about 2 minutes for medium rare, 3 minutes for medium, 4 minutes for medium-well and 5 minutes for well done.

Store the kebabs:

For saving your time in future, there is a hack you can do. Mix the minced lamb with all other ingredients and make a mixture. Now wrap the meat onto the bamboo skewers and place the skewers into a tray. Wrap the tray tightly with plastic wrap and store in refrigerator.

Vegetarian Ketogenic recipes

The list below includes the vegetarian ketogenic recipes that have no match in taste!

1- Low carb taco salad

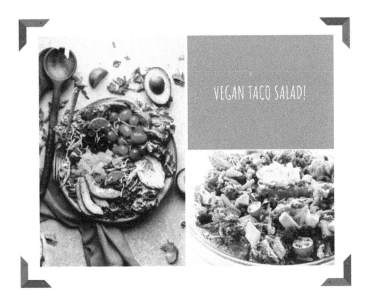

An easy recipe using common ingredients and can be ready in 20 minutes! A low carb keto salad that has no match in taste. It is naturally low in carbs, easy to prepare and absolutely delicious.

If you are a vegetarian, you will not find a better, richer in content salad than the keto taco salad. This crispy salad with a healthy mixture of cheese, purple onions, fresh tomatoes and creamy avocado.

There was a challenge making this meal a keto friendly because of the taco seasoning. Most of the taco seasoning available in the markets contain sugar or thickening corn starch that contain high carbs and eventually ruin the keto diet plan. So, finding a sugar-free taco seasoning remains a challenge. Whenever you buy a taco seasoning, make sure to read the sugar content in it!

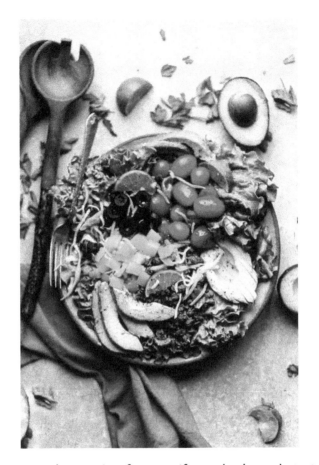

There is another option for you. If you don't get keto taco seasoning from the market, make it at your home using some common ingredients. Here is how to make it:

- ➢ 1 tsp chili powder
- ➢ 2 tsp cumin
- ➢ 1 tsp paprika
- ➢ 1 tsp garlic powder
- ➢ 1 tsp onion powder
- ➢ ½ tsp oregano
- ➢ ½ tsp black pepper

Above ingredients will make up 3 tsp of homemade taco seasoning and you don't need more than that for this recipe. You have an option to make it in a large quantity for future use.

Topping ideas:

There are a lot of topping ideas that can be used for topping taco salad. Here's the list and you can choose according to your choice.

- ➢ Sour cream
- ➢ Sliced black olives
- ➢ Pickled jalapenos
- ➢ Chopped cherry tomatoes
- ➢ Roasted bell peppers
- ➢ Crispy baked cheese

If you have a list of your own favorite toppings, go ahead and be creative to use them.

There was another challenge to make the taco salad suitable for vegetarians. Traditionally, taco salad contained ground beef in it so it was never a good choice for vegetarians.

We have got a solution for this. Replace the beef with cauliflower rice! This Taco salad with cauliflower is a vegetarian alternative. Meaty Cauliflower makes a great substitute for ground beef. Except for ground beef rest of the taco salad ingredients are totally unchanged. It has same flavor and texture.

Seasoned Cauliflower, fresh lettuce, crunchy veggies along with cheese, sour cream, and this salad is surely going to impress everyone.

Nutrition:

486 calories | 35g fats | 3g carbs | 34g proteins

Ingredients:

- 1 medium cauliflower
- Taco seasoning – ½ tsp
- Garlic powder – 1 tsp
- Chili powder – 1 tsp
- Salt as per taste
- Olive oil – 2tsp
- Fresh lemon juice – 1 tsp

For salad:

- Mixed salad leaves – 2 cups
- 1 Chopped onion
- Assorted pepper – 1 cup
- 1 avocado chopped
- Cherry tomatoes – 1 cup
- Shredded Cheddar cheese – 1 cup
- Fresh coriander leaves
- Sour cream

Instructions:

- In a bowl mix Olive Oil, Taco Seasoning, Garlic Powder, Chili Powder, salt. Add Cauliflower Florets and mix them well.

- Arrange seasoned cauliflower florets in a lined baking sheet. Bake in a pre-heated oven at 200°C for 20 minutes. Keep stirring to ensure even cooking.
- While Cauliflower ingredients are cooling down, in a big salad bowl add all the vegetables.
- Add cauliflower florets, shredded cheese, coriander leaves and mix them well. Serve immediately
- Top with sour cream and Tortilla Chips while serving.

2- <u>Avocado and Arugula Salad</u>

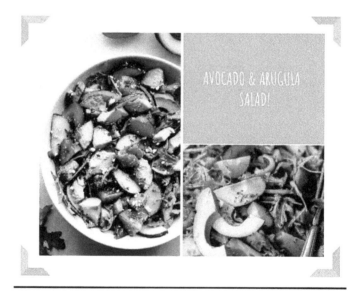

Simple and bright arugula salad with avocado, tomatoes, cucumbers, and shallots. A bright lemony vinaigrette with garlic and oregano brings it together. Peppery arugula with fresh cucumbers, juicy tomatoes, and creamy avocados. The perfect balance!

This is the quickest recipe to make. You just need to do some following cutting and chopping work before you start making the salad.

Cut the avocadoes into chunks, chop cucumbers into pieces without peeling them. Cut roma tomatoes into chunks, slice red onion. This is all the work that you have to do and the recipe will be ready automatically.

Is this salad healthy?

Most of the salads are healthy. As for this avocado salad, it is very helpful in fighting cancer, it is good for bones, reduces inflammation in body, cleanses the body and also avoids some neural disease. So, a delicious meal and a medicine package, all in one!

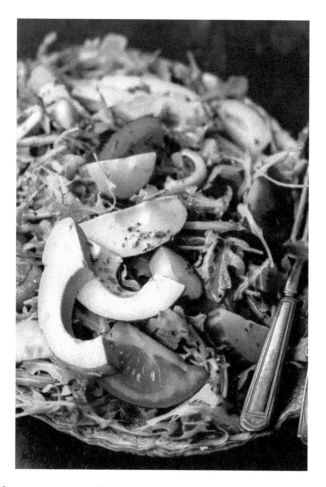

<u>Different possible variations:</u>

Following are the possible variations that you can do in order to enhance the taste and look of your avocado salad:

- ❖ Cheese: goat cheese or shaved parmesan instead of, or in addition to the feta cheese.
- ❖ Vegetables: carrots, broccoli, or cauliflower
- ❖ Nuts: pecans, walnuts or almonds

❖ Salad: mixed greens or spinach salad tastes good too.

You can add other ingredients that you love as well.

Nutrition:

219 kcal | 4g proteins | 19g fats | 6g carbs

Ingredients:

- 2 diced avocadoes
- 3 diced tomatoes
- 1 sliced cucumber
- Sliced red onion – ¼ cup
- Arugula – 1 cup
- Olive oil – 2 tsp
- Lemon juice – 2 tsp
- Feta cheese – ¼ cup
- Salt and pepper

Instructions:

- In a large bowl combine avocado, cucumber, tomatoes, red onion and arugula. Gently toss.
- In a small bowl whisk the olive oil, and lemon juice. Add to the veggies and toss.
- Serve with crumbled feta cheese.

Note:

Eat the fresh salad, do not store for future use as the vegetables will become acidic.

3- Shaved Fennel and Celery Salad

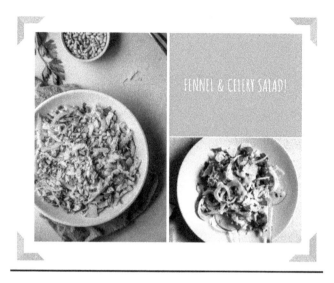

Enjoy the texture and freshness of this salad alongside a nice potato pancake and a soft-cooked egg

The richly nutritious and low carb keto salad that will make your day. The vegetarians have got nothing to worry when they have Shaved Fennel and celery salad on their lunch table. This Shaved Fennel and Celery Salad comes together quickly and has such a delicious light lemon vinaigrette and wonderful crunch. It's the perfect side salad for rich and hearty dishes like pasta or braised short ribs.

Its crunchiness, its tanginess, its easiness, its taste, its looks Oh! These all would make you feel happy and fresh all the day.

This fennel and celery salad is so fresh and bright and crunchy. The little bits of celery and sharp fennel blend so nicely with the light citrus dressing, and that shaved Parmesan and the toasted pine nuts add a wonderful buttery, nuttiness.

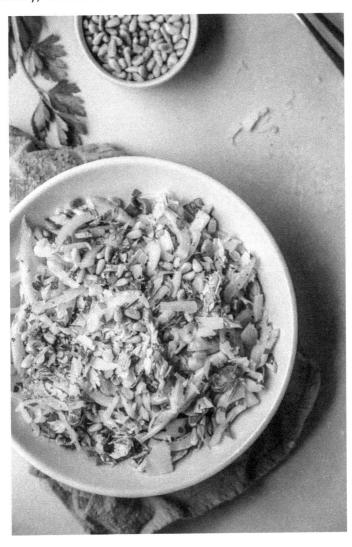

This salad is also great because you can make it ahead of time, which means it's perfect for bringing to a potluck or packing along for lunches. I would say that the taste is best the day you make it, but it still maintains its crunchy bite for a few days. If you'd like to make it way in advance, say a few days prior, I would just reserve the lemon juice and olive oil and toss that in at the end.

Nutrition:

221 kcal | 4g Carbs | 7g Proteins | 20g Fats

Ingredients:

- Pine nuts – ¼ cup
- Thinly sliced fennel bulb – 1 large
- Chopped parsley – ½ cup
- Olive oil – 3 tsp
- Shaved parmesan – ¼ cup
- Thinly sliced celery stalks – 5
- Lemon juice – ¼ cup

Instructions:

- Take a pan or skillet and heat over low to medium heat by adding pine nuts. Toast the nuts for 5-10 minutes until they become goldish brown in color. Keep a check on the nuts so that they may not get burnt.
- Take a bowl and add thinly sliced fennel and celery. Also add chopped parsley into it.
- Mix the fennel, celery and parsley with oil and fresh lemon juice. Sprinkle salt and pepper over it as required.

- Now pour shaved parmesan and toasted pine nuts over the salad and enjoy the taste.

Note:

- This salad retains its great crunch for a couple of days, so be sure to save any leftovers!
- Store any leftover pine nuts in the freezer - They'll stay fresh for much longer this way.

4- Ketogenic Cauliflower rice

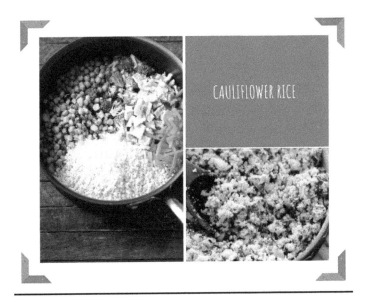

This Keto Cauliflower Rice, Bell Pepper, Parsley and Feta Salad is a versatile side dish that can be enjoyed either hot or cold!

This dish is mostly used as a side dish but due to its taste and nutrition's, we are going to make it the main dish for your lunch table.

Cauliflower rice itself is a simple dish but it opens doors to a whole heaven of toppings and variations that you can try on it. It can bear any kind of topping and that is beauty of this dish. You can add cream cheese, mint leaves, mint sauce, red chili sauce, seasoned tacos, mushrooms, vegetables, beans, peanuts, almond, walnut and a lot more as toppings. You just need to imagine and be creative, then see the magical taste and look of this dish. It is going to be the delicious meal today!

When we talk about a keto meal, we are not only concerned about the taste of the dish but also the health aspects linked with that dish. In case of this dish, you need not to worry! You will not find a keto friendly dish than this in any other kind of diet.

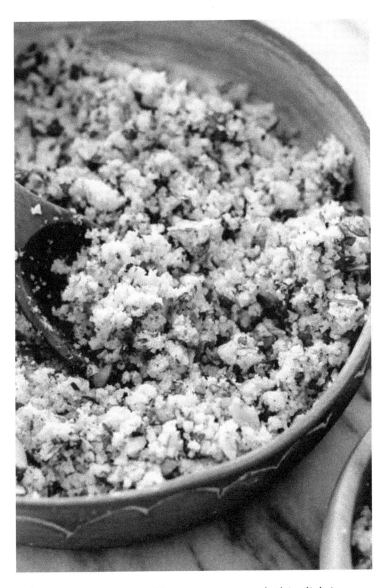

When it comes to cooking, you can cook this dish in your beloved style. You may cook it in Greek style or you may like to make it simple to save your time. You've got options, so let your imagination add taste into it!

You may consider make it by roasting it. Roasting takes cauliflower to a level of tasty that far surpasses any other way of cooking it. Steaming is ok, but for this you REALLY need to roast it in the olive oil and garlic before adding all the tasty antipasto accompaniments. You could use store bought cauliflower rice and add in some olive oil and garlic to season it and this would certainly save some time, but I prefer the oven roasting method if you have time.

Nutrition:

132 kcal | 6g protein | 5g carbs | 9g fats

Ingredients:

- Cauliflower florets – 8 cups
- Olive oil – 3 tsp
- Mozzarella smoked and chopped – 4 ounces
- Roasted red pepper – 6 ounces
- Banana pepper rings -1 ounce
- Sliced olives – ½ cup
- Basil chopped – 1 cup
- Vinegar – 3 tsp
- Salt and pepper to taste

Instructions:

- Pre-heat oven to 370-400°F. Place cauliflower florets on baking pan and add olive oil into it.
- Bake for 50-60 minutes then place the baked cauliflower florets into a food processor and pulse until texture of rice.

- Now cook the cauliflower rice in a large skillet tossing with the olive oil until warmed and then follow the rest of recipe.
- Now pour the rice into a bowl and allow to cool.
- Once cooled, add other remaining ingredients into the bowl and mix together.
- Sprinkle salt and pepper to taste and enjoy the dish.

Note:

Store the leftover for future use, freeze it or take it in a plastic wrap box for eating during traveling etc.

5- Ketogenic cauliflower potato salad

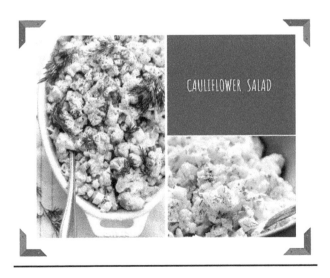

This quick & easy cauliflower mock potato salad recipe is low carb, keto, paleo, gluten-free, whole 30, and healthy. It's a crowd pleaser for everyone, too!

The cauliflower taste is actually quite mild, and the texture is very much like regular potato salad. The key is cooking the cauliflower to the same softness as cooked potatoes would be. Make sure your florets are very small, too. This low carb potato salad is just like the one you're probably used to. It has the classic add-ins of celery, and onions. The dressing is your typical mayonnaise base with mustard, vinegar (apple cider to keep it paleo!), and spices. So simple, and so good.

While cauliflower might not be your first choice when you think of a real potato salad, in the low carb world, cauliflower is the veggie most likely to replace potato. The texture and bite of tender cauliflower can resemble the texture and bite of potato salad, although the taste is obviously not the same. The end result though can make a traditional high carb recipe, much lower in carbs and just as satisfying. Should you expect it to taste like potato? Absolutely not. It is cauliflower, but the dressing will bring you back to the potato salad you might have enjoyed prior to going low carb.

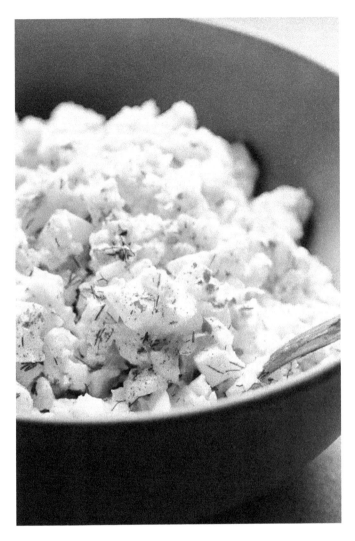

Nutrients:

227 kcal | 20g Fats | 7g carbs | 5g protein

Ingredients:

- Cauliflower – 1 pound
- Mayonnaise – 1/3 cup

- Olive oil – 1 tsp
- White vinegar – 2 tsp
- Garlic powder – 1tsp
- Paprika – ¼ tsp
- Celery salt – ¼ tsp
- Pepper and salt – as required
- Sliced red onion – ¼ cup
- Chopped scallions – ¼ cup
- Garlic powder – 1 tsp
- Dijon mustard – 1 tsp

Instructions:

- Steam the cauliflower until fork tender, about 10 minutes. Cool to room temperature for 20-30 minutes.
- Whisk the other ingredients together, taste and adjust salt if needed.
- Stir the dressing in the bowl with the cauliflower then add in the onion and scallions.
- Chill for 30 minutes or until ready to serve.

Ketogenic dinner recipes

If you are in a wonder that what you will make for dinner that will be low carb and keto friendly then take yourself out of this wonder. How is it possible that ketogenic diet after providing breakfast and lunch recipes would leave it totally over you to make your dinner! A complete list of keto friendly dinner recipes is going to be in your hands.

Non-vegetarian recipes

1- Creamy Tuscan garlic chicken

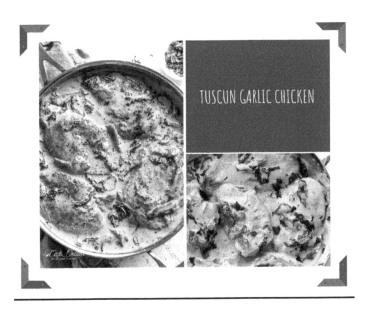

What is Tuscan style chicken?

When you season chicken breasts or thighs with Italian herbs, you have made a Tuscan style chicken. This seasoned chicken is then served in garlic cream sauce with parmesan cheese. You may also add Gouda cheese in it. Adding fresh spinach leaves and tomatoes in cream sauce is also an option.

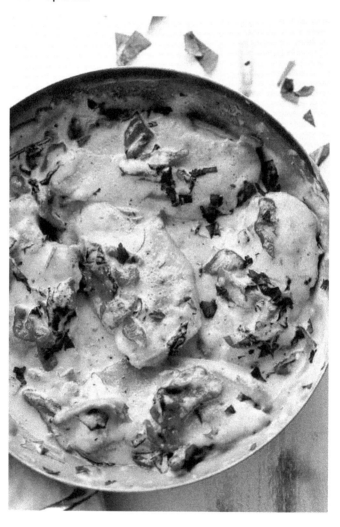

What are Italian herbs?

Some typical Italian herbs are:

- ➢ Dried basil
- ➢ Crushed rosemary
- ➢ Dried thyme
- ➢ Sage
- ➢ Fennel seeds

If you have got no problem with spices, then you should consider blending spices to make quick sauce to enhance the flavor of recipe. But if you are not fine with having spices, no worries, you can simply make less spicy or spice-free sausage as well. You can also add onion or garlic powder as well if you like.

Making Tuscan chicken a few hours ahead:

If you want to make this meal a few hours ahead of time or even the night before, follow the directions as you normally would but when searing the chicken, remove it when its internal temperature reaches 155-160 degrees F. Since the internal temperature of chicken should be 165 degrees F, undercooking the chicken a little will keep you from overcooking the chicken when you reheat it later on.

Then, about 30 minutes before you're ready to eat, cover with tin-foil and place the entire oven-proof skillet or cast iron pan in the oven and bake at 350 degrees F until the chicken reaches 165 degrees F.

Servings:

Now, we must talk about what can we serve with Keto Tuscan chicken? What you say about zucchini noodles? Yes a great option. Serve the Tuscan chicken with zucchini noodles. Serving with pasta is also an option but it is high carb so the balance would be lost. Serving with roasted cauliflower rice would also be a great option. You may also consider beans as servings with Tuscan chicken. As it pleases you, if you have any other idea, go for it but be careful about carbs. Because the sausage is already rich, so adding a few more carbs will not be a right choice.

Nutrition:

524 kcal | 4g carbs | 44g proteins | 37g fats

Ingredients:

- Olive oil – 2 tsp
- Boneless skinless chicken breast – 2 ¼ lbs
- Minced garlic – 4 cloves
- Italian seasoning – ½ tsp
- Paprika – ½ tsp
- Butter – 2 tsp
- Heavy cream – 1 ¼ cup
- Parmesan cheese – ½ cup
- Grated gouda cheese – 1/3 cup
- Grape Tomatoes – 1 cup
- Chopped onion – ¼
- Spinach leaves – 1 ½ cup

Instructions:

- Season chicken with Italian seasoning, paprika, salt and pepper.
- In a 12-inch cast-iron skillet over medium heat, add 2 tbsp olive oil.
- When the skillet gets nice and hot, add your chicken and sear on both sides until brown. Put a lid on the top to help the chicken cook. Don't overcook the chicken. The internal temperature should reach 165°F. (Use a thermometer to help.) Remove from the pan and set aside.
- Add butter, garlic, onion, and diced tomatoes to pan with Italian seasoning and paprika sauce for 5 minutes stirring occasionally on medium/ low heat.
- De-glaze pan with chicken broth. Scrape the pan to remove the bits that might have stuck to the bottom. Make sure to keep them in the pan as they add incredible flavor.
- Add heavy cream, Parmesan cheese, Gouda, and spinach and simmer on medium heat until the sauce begins to thicken stirring occasionally so that it doesn't stick. (It took mine approx. seven minutes.)
- Add the chicken back to the skillet, and simmer on low heat for two minutes.
- Add remaining 1/4 cup of Parmesan cheese on top of chicken if desired.

Note:

- If you want to fry your chicken better and want to get better flavor then use cast-iron skillet.
- Use full-fat heavy cream
- Gouda cheese is an optional ingredient, but do consider it for a better flavor.
- Sun-dried tomatoes instead of fresh tomatoes may also be used.

2- Keto grilled Mediterranean chicken salad

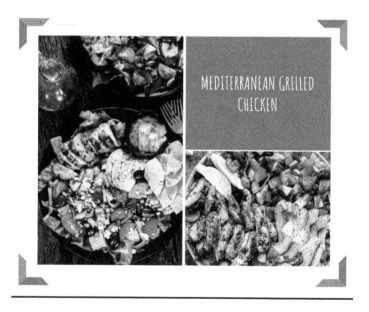

A quick, easy, full of flavor and low carb diet that will please your eyes with its looks too! Juicy marinated chicken with homemade vinegar and oil dressing makes this dish similar to Horiatiki.

If you marinate the chicken in vinegar or lemon juice, olive oil, garlic, thyme, salt and pepper, it will give the chicken a lot of tasty flavor. An hour marinating will be enough. If you want to skip marinating process then you can make the chicken in 'Slow cooker' recipe style but it will take more time so marinating is recommended.

Once the chicken is marinated, you can cook it in more than one ways. You may consider cooking the chicken in a skillet or pan. It's the easiest way. Just heat the skillet containing olive oil over flame. Add chicken and cook for five minutes, then change the side and again cook for five minutes and you have your chicken ready.

The other way is grilling. It takes about 5 to 15 minutes to grill chicken. You can also bake the chicken in a pre-heated oven for 25- 35 minutes.

It depends on you how you want to cook the chicken for the best desired taste.

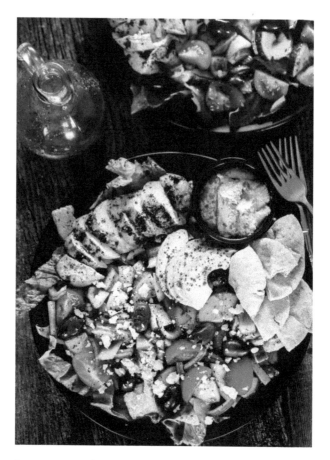

Some important tips:

- Use the FULL marinate time, it will make a big difference in the finished flavor of the salad.
- When using a skillet to cook the chicken make sure it's properly hot so you get a great finish on your chicken.
- If you want to change up the salad vegetables you can swap them out for any others you prefer.
- Extra vinaigrette dressing can be kept it in the fridge for later.

Making the salad ahead of time:

You can make this dish head of time. You just need to cook the chicken and prepare the vegetables to make dressing ahead of time. When it's time to serve, you can assemble the salad and serve.

Nutrition:

14g carbs | 24g proteins | 269 kcal | 39g fats

Ingredients:

- Arugula – 2 cups
- Baby spinach – 2 cups
- Cucumber – ½
- Olives – ¾ cup
- Sliced red onion – 2 ounces
- 1 sliced avocado
- Romaine lettuce – 2 cups
- Cherry tomatoes – 1 cup
- Sliced basil leaves (optional)
- Mozzarella cheese (option) – 1cup

For marinating chicken:

- Bone less Chicken thighs – 4 pieces
- Lemon zest
- Lemon juice – 2tsp
- Olive oil – 2 tsp
- Crushed garlic – 4 cloves
- Fresh thyme leaves – 1 tsp
- Salt – 1 tsp
- Pepper – ½ tsp

- Balsamic vinegar – 2 tsp
- Dijon mustard – 1 tsp

Instructions:

- Mix the chicken with marinating ingredients and marinate the chicken for one hour.
- After marinating, cook the chicken by grilling it or cook it in a skillet or bake in oven.
- Take a bowl and whisk all the ingredients until the oil and vinegar are combined.
- Assemble the Mediterranean chicken salad by adding arugula, baby spinach leaves, avocado, sliced grilled chicken, tomatoes, cucumber, olives, red onion and cheese (optional).
- Pour the salad dressing and sprinkle salt and pepper to taste.

3- Cauliflower rice with chicken meatballs

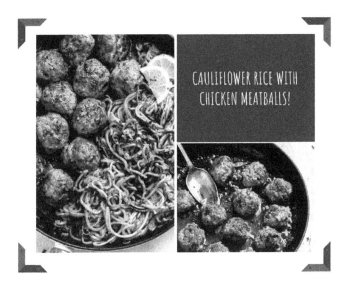

Few things are as satisfying as juicy, tender meatballs. They put all of our cravings to rest because, well, they're usually an indulgence. So we created a leaner dish that doesn't sacrifice any flavor: Whole30 chicken meatballs and cauliflower rice with creamy coconut-herb sauce. Sound like a mouthful? That's because it is, in the best way possible.

The meatballs would take traditional keto cauliflower rice to another level. Gently simmered in tomato sauce, these meat balls can beautifully complement the cauliflower rice.

When it comes to cook meat balls, there are two opinions. You may like to pan fry the meat balls, yes it is a good idea it will surely add into the flavor of the dish but the meatballs will not maintain their round shape. Another opinion is baking meatballs, if you bake the meatballs, their shape will remain round. There is another creative option that you may consider, you can partially bake the meatballs for their round shape and then pan fry them. This will give you a good round and flavor meat balls. Depends on you, which way you want to make them.

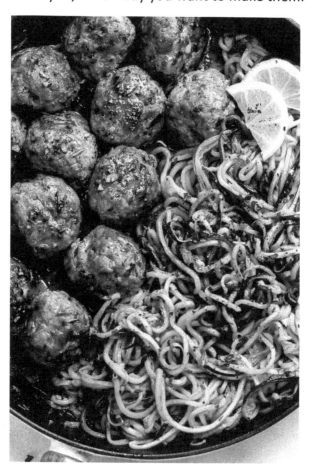

Traditionally, paste of bread or bread crumbs are used to make the meatballs juicy but it also makes the dish high carb. Yes, it is for sure that everyone wants juicy meatballs but ingredients must be low carb. You've got a very beautiful idea to make meatballs juicy in a keto friendly way is to use heavy cream. This will add moisture and fats both to your meat balls.

Extra cheese holds these tender meatballs together perfectly without any type of flour. A breeze to whip up makes these the perfect weeknight dinner for everyone.

A great keto meal for those who want to avoid carbs and also want a taste that has got no match. This dish with a crisp salad with squeezed lemon juice is a greatly tasty dish you have ever eaten.

Ingredients:

- Olive oil (extra-virgin) – 1 tsp
- Red onion – ½
- Minced garlic – 2 cloves
- Ground chicken – 1 pound
- Crumbled chicken bouillon – 1
- Chicken broth – ½ cup
- Italian seasoning (optional) – 1 tsp
- Chopped fresh parsley – ¼ cup
- Ground black pepper – ½ tsp

For sauce:

- Coconut milk – 14 ounce
- Chopped fresh parsley – 1 ¼ cups
- Roughly chopped scallions – 4

- 1 garlic clove
- Lemon zest and juice
- Cauliflower rice – 1 serving

Instructions:

- Make cauliflower rice with a large grater or food processor. Transfer to a shallow plate with 1/2 cup water and cook covered in the microwave for 4 minutes.
- In the meantime, in a large bowl, combine ground chicken, cheese, grated garlic, Italian seasoning, crumbled bouillon cube, red chili pepper flakes, chopped cilantro, and black pepper. Mix well with your hands or fork and form medium balls. Arrange on a plate and set aside.
- Melt 2 tablespoons butter in a large skillet over medium-low heat. Cook the chicken meatballs for 8 – 10 minutes on all sides, until browned and cooked through. While cooking, baste the meatballs with the mix of butter and juices. Remove to a clean plate and set aside.
- In the same skillet melt remaining tablespoon butter; then add lemon juice, chicken stock, hot sauce, minced garlic, parsley and red pepper flakes (if you want). Cook for 3 or 4 minutes, stirring regularly until the sauce has reduced a bit. Adjust seasoning with salt and pepper and garnish with more cilantro or parsley if you like.
- Divide cauliflower rice into meal prep containers. Then top with chicken meatballs and garnish with lemon slices. Drizzle a little of the sauce over the

meatballs and cauliflower rice, or keep the sauce into small containers. Reheat quickly in the microwave when ready to heat. Enjoy!

4- <u>Tasty Keto zucchini slice</u>

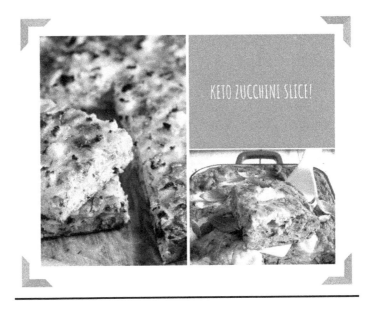

This keto Zucchini Slice is a popular lunchbox classic except ours is very low carb! It is an ideal lunch or cheesy snack that everyone loves.

The keto zucchini slice is easily customized to your tastes, add a 1/2 cup of cooked bacon to make it meatier, or add 3 tablespoons of your favorite herbs to boost the flavor.

A zucchini is a thin-skinned cultivar of what in Britain and Ireland is referred to as a marrow. In South Africa, zucchini is known as baby marrow. Along with certain other squashes and pumpkins, the zucchini belongs to the species Cucurbit pepo. The zucchini is treated as a vegetable; it is usually cooked and presented as a savory dish or accompaniment. Botanically, zucchinis are fruits, a type of botanical berry called a "pepo", being the swollen ovary of the zucchini flower.

Traditionally, recipe doesn't include many vegetables, but sky is the limit for you if you are in the kitchen. You can add variations and prepare tasty and yummy toppings as well. You can add your favorite herbs, Italian seasoning, or bacon as well. Sprinkle black pepper as topping and feel the fragrance.

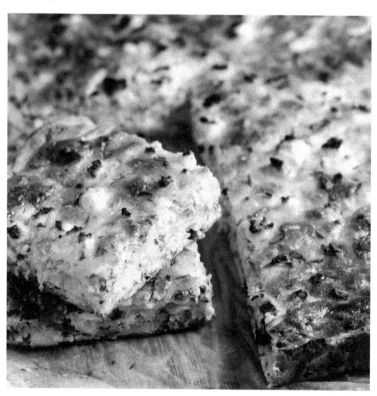

Instead of starchy bread crumbs or corn flour, you will use keto friendly almond flour in this recipe. Almond flour is low carb keto friendly flour and it adds into the taste a lot.

This Recipe will make 25 snack serves for you. You have got an option to store the zucchini slices in the fridge for future use. They can be used up to 5 days.

Nutrition:

8g fats | 2g carbs | 4g protein | 76 kcal per serving

Zucchini slice Ingredients:

- Salted butter – 1 tsp
- Diced Onion – 1 small
- Crushed Garlic – 2 cloves
- 2 large Zucchini – 600g
- Roughly chopped zucchini Baby spinach – 2 ounces
- Shredded Cheddar cheese – ½ cup
- Feta cheese - ½ cup
- Almond flour – 1 cup
- Baking powder – 1 tsp
- Salt – 1 tsp
- 5 large eggs
- Heavy cream – ¼ cup

Instructions:

- Keep your oven temperate to 180°c or 350°F.
- Take a saucepan and put butter onion and garlic in it. Cook them a little over medium heat until the onion is translucent.

- Place the grated zucchini coarsely, place into a clean towel and squeeze out as much liquid as you can.
- Now take a bowl and add onion mixture, spinach, and cheddar cheese, half of feta cheese, almond flour, baking powder, salt and pepper along with the squeezed zucchini and mix them together well.
- Now add eggs and cream and whisk.
- Line the baking pan with parchment paper and pour zucchini mixture into it and smooth out evenly.
- Pour the remaining half feta cheese over the mixture and bake for 20-35 minutes until golden brown.
- Then take the baking pan out and let it cool for 15 minutes before cutting into servings.

Note:

- **Store or refrigerate the leftover for future use.**
- **Cut into the pieces (slices), put into the plastic wrap or box and take it along you and enjoy while you are in bus or train.**

5- <u>Ketogenic pan-seared steaks with mushrooms</u>

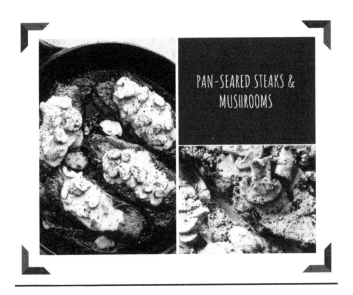

This recipe is one of the must-have recipes for all meat lovers. What's better than a dinner table having seared steaks with delicious toppings during your keto diet? This recipe is highly keto friendly and has a whole universe of variations that you can try with it.

So, the main ingredient for these recipes is meat. It is recommended that you buy boneless steaks that are around 1 or 1.5 inch thick as well. As we are preparing a ketogenic meal so it must contain more fat, so thick steaks are preferred to increase the fat content in recipe.

Moreover, this fat in thick steaks will help in making the steaks juicy when you will cook it. Make sure you buy antibiotics and hormones – free meat so that your health may not be affected.

Now we come to the ways of cooking this delicious recipe. As clear from the name of recipe, you are going to sear the meat in pan. The taste of your steak will be dependent on temperature and time you cook it over flame. So there are options and you have to choose which one suits you the best.

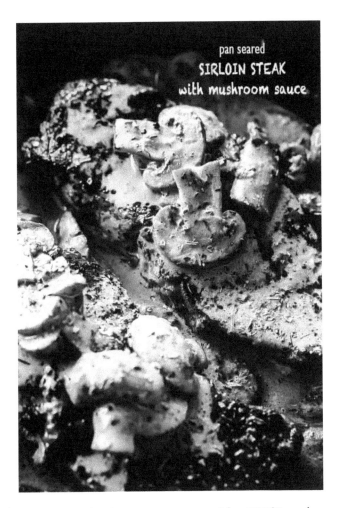

pan seared
SIRLOIN STEAK
with mushroom sauce

- ➤ Rare steak: Temperature must be 125°F and cooking time must be 5-6 minutes. But this method is not recommended for most of the people yet there are people who would like it this way)
- ➤ Medium rare steak: Cook your steak for 6-8 minutes with temperature 130°F
- ➤ Medium steak: Cook steak for 9-10 minutes with 140°F temperature.
- ➤ Well done steak: 160°F and 12 minutes of cooking.

Best way to keep a check on temperature is using thermometer.

Some Tips:

- ➤ Before starting cooking, make sure to keep your steaks at room temperature. You can do this by removing steaks from refrigerator about 30-60 minutes prior to cooking.
- ➤ Make sure to place the mushrooms in pan in single layer, this will give them a crispy brown look.
- ➤ Pat dry the steaks using towel paper. This will help the steaks to get brown crust.
- ➤ As the meat is going to cook very fast, so you should have all the ingredients and thermometer handy.
- ➤ Before searing the meat, season it with coarse salt for about 30 minutes. It will create a nice dry surface to sear the meat.
- ➤ Don't use spices like black pepper during searing the meat, because the pan will be very hot and the pepper may burn and ruin the taste and fragrance of meat.

Nutrition:

411 kcal | 35g fat | 6g carbs | 20g protein

Ingredients:

- • Extra virgin olive oil – 1 tsp
- • Mushrooms – 6 ounces
- • Butter – 1 tsp
- • Minced Garlic – 3 cloves

- Salt and pepper to taste

For making steak:

- Lean strip steaks – 2
- Coarse salt
- Smashed garlic – 3 cloves
- Fresh thyme springs – 3
- Grass-fed butter – 3 tsp

Instructions:

- Keep the steaks in room temperature for about 30-60 minutes prior cooking. Pat dry the steaks using paper towel.
- Season all sides of steaks with coarse salt and let marinate a little bit.
- Take a pan or skillet and put over medium flame. Add olive oil and butter and sauté mushrooms, garlic and salt. Cook for about 3 minutes and set aside in a plate.
- Now increase the flame to high and let the pan heat up for about 2-3 minutes until the pan smokes a bit.
- Now place the steaks in the hot skillet and cook for about 2 minutes each side. Let the steaks get a nice crust.
- Now add other ingredients like butter, garlic and thyme into the skillet and tilt the skillet to spread the butter.

- Now use spoon to pour the butter in the skillet over the steaks. Flip the steaks and check their internal temperature. When the steaks are cooked to your desired temperature, bring the mushrooms and serve hot. It will increase the dish's look if you serve it with roasted green beans, asparagus cauliflower.

Ketogenic dinner recipes for Vegetarians

1- <u>Keto Broccoli Cheddar Soup</u>

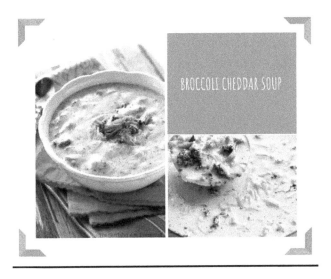

A keto friendly and vegetarian friendly soup that is creamy, delicious and very low carb. Let me clear one thing in the beginning. This soup is not too thick because it doesn't contain thickening agents or starchy ingredients. You might be used to thick soups, but taste this thinner soup once and you will forget those thick soups. Use different ingredients or herbs to bring creative flavors to your dish.

There are more than a million recipes to make broccoli soup but they lack one and the most important thing and that is 'low carb content'. These recipes mostly use thickening agents like flour and other starchy ingredients. This recipe is going to give you a starch-free, low carb broccoli cheddar soup in matters of 20 minutes or so!

The beauty of this soup lies in the fact that it is not just for those people who are following a diet plan. It is for anyone who wants to taste something different and anyone who tastes it falls in love with it. This soup is completely a healthy diet and is considered clean eating.

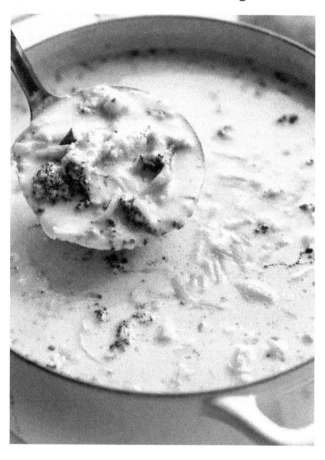

If you are finding the easiest recipe of soup to make very easily and in less time than you have come to the right place. This vegetarian, healthy soup is probably one of the easiest recipes to make. Just a few simple ingredients and a few minutes, here is your soup ready!

Some tips:

- Avoid too high heat while cooking this recipe to avoid seizing and sticking.
- The more broccolis you leave in before pureeing, the thicker your broccoli soup will be. The cheese helps thicken your broccoli cheddar soup, but the pureed broccoli florets will, too!
- Use immersion blender to puree the broccoli along with cheddar cheese into the soup.
- If you want to cook your soup more quickie, you can use frozen broccoli.

Some fantastic variations:

Once you have mastered the basic process, there comes the time to do some tasty variations.

You can consider following ingredients as extras for your soup.

- Your favorite spices or Italian seasoning
- Cauliflower, bell peppers and onions
- Cooked bacon
- Sun dried tomatoes

The possibilities are endless, just let your imagination and creativity do magic for you!

Nutrients:

292 kcal | 25g fat | 5g carbs | 13g protein

Ingredients:

- Broccoli (Cut into florets) – 4 cups
- Minced garlic – 4 cloves
- Vegetable broth – 3 ½ cups
- Heavy cream – 1 cup
- Shredded cheddar cheese – 3 cups

Instructions:

- Take a pan and sauté garlic in it for about 1-2 minutes.
- Add heavy cream, chopped broccoli and vegetable broth into the pan and heat to boil. Cook for about 10-20 minutes until the broccoli is tender.
- **Option 1**: If you want to follow the original way then add shredded cheddar cheese gradually stirring constantly until melted. Make sure to keep heat very low otherwise it may seize. Take it out of the heat immediately when it has melted.
- **Option 2**: This method is recommended for better taste. Remove about 1/3 of the broccoli pieces using a slotted spoon and set aside. Use an immersion blender to puree the remaining broccoli. Then add shredded cheddar cheese ½ cup at a time over low heat. Stir it continuously until melted and smooth.
- Remove from the heat and put the reserved broccoli florets back to the soup.

- Cook the recipe the way you want, then dress it with cooked bacon or other vegetables and enjoy the meal!

2- Cheese shell taco cups

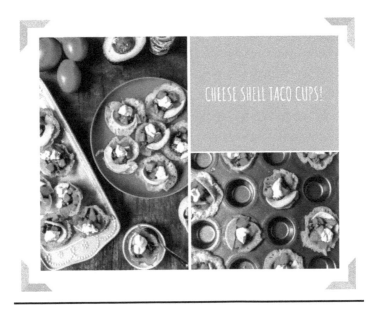

The ultimate keto recipe, taco shells made out of crispy cheese. Baking little mounds of cheddar cheese and shaping them into hand held cups. This fun option recipe for those who are following keto diet and want something really fun and quick! These easy cheese taco shells are perfect for making keto Tacos! Baked cheddar cheese formed into the shape of a taco and filled with seasoned ground beef for a low carb taco night!

This is basically a Mexican recipe, low in carbs and rich in fats! These taco shells are gluten-free and easy to make and for sure they taste more than the original tacos.

So, here comes a question that how to make the tacos from cheese? Here is your answer.

Use a baking sheet with parchment paper or silicon mat to line the piles of grated cheese.

Place thee baking sheet in oven and bake for 5-8 minutes at 350°F, until the shredded cheese melts and edges become brown. It's important to wait until those edges start to get crispy because you'll get the crispiest cheese taco shells that way.

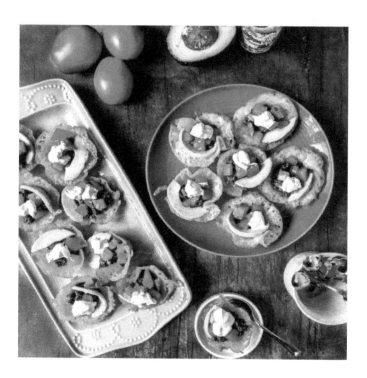

Use two glasses and sit a thick handled spoon across the glasses. You'll want the handle to be thick enough that it will leave a space of about 3/4" in the curve of your taco. It doesn't have to be precise! Let the cheese cool for a minute then lift it off of the baking sheet and drape it over the spoon handle. Let it cool completely, this only takes about 5 minutes, and you have a low carb taco shell!

Nutrition:

261 kcal | 2g carbs |17g protein |21g fats

Ingredients:

- Shredded Cheddar cheese – 2 cups
- Homemade taco seasoning – 2 tsp
- Water – ¼ cup
- Toppings for taco
- Sour cream, Avocado, Cheese (Optional)

Instructions:

- Preheat the oven to 350°F. Take a baking sheet with parchment paper or a silicone mat and line with 1/4 cup piles of cheese 2 inches apart. Press the cheese down lightly to make one layer.
- Place baking sheet in the oven and bake for 5-7 minutes until the cheese turns brown.
- Let the cheese cool for 1-2 minutes in room temperature until it is firm enough to lift but still bendable. Balance a spoon or a rod shaped utensil

on two cups and place the cheese over the handle. Let cheese cool completely then remove.

- Add the homemade taco seasoning in a pan and cook for a while. Add other ingredients into the pan and mix well. Pour water into skillet and stir everything together.
- Cook for 5 minutes until liquid (Water) has evaporated.
- Serve taco shells and top with your favorite taco toppings.
- Here is the meal ready. Enjoy your meal!

3- <u>Gluten-Free Cheese and Cauliflower 'Breadsticks'</u>

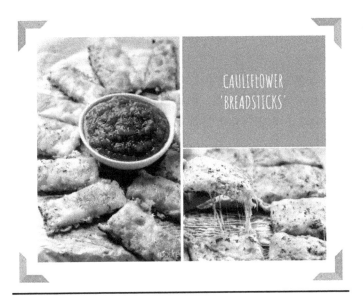

A dish from heavens. What else you need if you have a vegetarian friendly, keto friendly, low carb, high fats, deliciously tasty and amazingly dressed everything in one plate. Yes, this gluten-free cheese and cauliflower breadsticks recipe is going to take your keto diet to another level. You'll love how easy it is to make these cheesy cauliflower breadsticks! They're the perfect finger food to serve at parties, or whip up a batch when you need a tasty, satisfying snack.

Making Cauliflower breadsticks:

It is a very simple task. You don't need to buy readymade breadsticks from store. You can easily make them at home.

You just need to add the cauliflower into the food processor and pulse it a few times until it becomes like rice. Then microwave the processed cauliflower for about 10 minutes. Add eggs and cheese along with your favorite spices and shape it into your crust. That's all you have to do!

There is no need to squeeze water or anything like that. You need not to worry about that, you have already got a nice firm crust. This is the easiest way of doing this task.

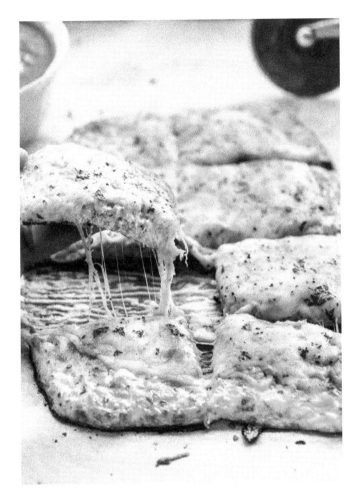

Making pizza crust with this recipe:

If you want to have pizza on your dinner table instead of breadsticks, this recipe gives you the option too! You can make pizza crust instead of making breadsticks out of processed cauliflower. You need to follow the same process of making crust as above and then top the crust with pizza sauce and other toppings and here is you pizza ready.

Making crust without microwave:

So if you don't have a microwave, it is recommended that you cook the cauliflower first in an oven or over stove before processing in food processor. Rest of the process is similar as explained above.

What if cauliflower is soggy after microwaving?

After microwaving, your cauliflower shouldn't be soggy. But in case it is, just put it on few paper towels and squeeze it to drain out water.

One more beautiful thing about cauliflower crust is that it doesn't fall apart when you pick up a slice or breadstick for eating. It is a firm crust and cheese holds it tight.

These Cheesy Cauliflower Breadsticks are gluten free, low carb and so delicious! Use this crust for breadsticks or for pizza. This recipe is a winner and a keeper!

Nutrition:

174 kcal | 4g carbs | 13g proteins | 11g Fats

Ingredients:

- Riced Cauliflower – 4 cups
- Mozzarella cheese – 3 cups
- Oregano – 3 tsp
- Minced garlic – 4 cloves
- Salt and pepper to taste

Instructions:

- Preheat oven to 420 to 425°. Line the baking sheet with parchment paper.
- Chop the cauliflower into florets. Add the florets to your food processor and pulse few times until cauliflower becomes like rice.
- Place the cauliflower in a microwave and microwave for about 10 minutes. Remove the cauliflower from microwave and let it cool until all the steam goes out. Place the microwaved cauliflower in a large bowl and 2 cups of mozzarella, oregano, garlic, salt and pepper. Mix all the ingredients well.
- Take two baking sheets and separate the mixture into two halves. Put each half on a separate sheet and shape the crust in either pizza crust or breadsticks according to your choice.
- Bake the crust without topping for about 25 – 30 minutes until the crust becomes golden. Then take the crust out and sprinkle mozzarella cheese and Bake again for another 5-7 minutes until the cheese is melted and set.
- Now top the dish with your favorite spices and seasonings and enjoy the meal!

Note:

- If you don't have microwave, cook the cauliflower a little bit before processing in food processor.
- Do not process the cauliflower too much otherwise the crust will not be firm.

- The cauliflower should not be soggy at all after microwaving it. If however, you find that it is soggy, place it on a few paper towels and squeeze the water out of it.

4- <u>Low-Carb Lasagna Stuffed Spaghetti Squash</u>

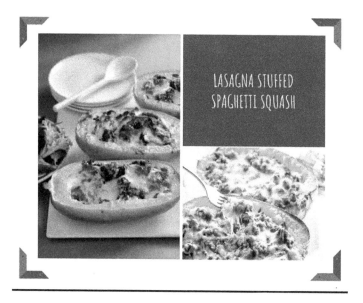

A low carb, vegetarian friendly and delicious meal. This meal is going to be one of your favorite meals after you taste it once. If you are looking for healthy dish that also tastes great and is keto friendly as well, this is the right recipe for you. Lasagna stuffed spaghetti squash is ultimately healthy, low carb and delicious meal that is going to make your keto days full of taste.

This recipe can be considered an ultimate resolve if to be cooked unplanned. There may come a time to you when guests arrive suddenly and you have nothing to prepare except some common ingredients in your kitchen. No worries, you can convert those common ingredients into a lovely and magically delicious dish that also looks a lot special and your guests will think that you prepared something very special for them. For a quickie, you will just need ingredients like olive oil, sea salt, black pepper, garlic, Italian seasoning and cheese. These are the common ingredients and are mostly present in kitchen especially if you are following a ketogenic diet.

But if you have time and there is no emergency, then you can surely give this dish an unmatched taste. In this case, you should use three cheeses namely ricotta, parmesan and mozzarella. Moreover, you can add anything that you can imagine. Sky is the limit for you!

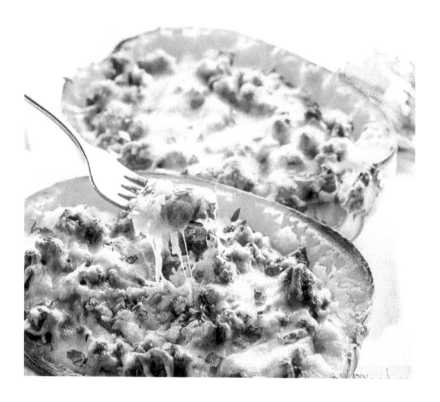

You will need to buy spaghetti squash. This one is the only ingredient that you may not have already presented in your kitchen. You will need to go to a store near buy and look for it.

To add an extra taste into your dish, you ay like to consider the marinara sauce and Italian seasoning. This sauce suits best with this dish. You can easily find the sauce in the store but make sure to buy sugar-free. If you don't find one, you can make at home as well and it will not be a much complicated task.

Yummy layers:

Spaghetti squash lasagna boats basically have three layers. These layers include cheesy parmesan ricotta spaghetti squash, Italian or any other seasoning and melted mozzarella. You have got two options for the first layer. You can keep spaghetti squash strands separate from parmesan and ricotta. And you can also mix them. It is tasty both ways and you can consider the option you want. But yes, it tastes better when the spaghetti squash layer is cheesy. Simply make each layer according to the instructions, and store in glass containers in the fridge. When you are ready to serve, assemble the spaghetti squash boats and heat in the oven.

You could also do the assembly ahead of time if you wanted to. But, the downside is that the seasoning may seep through the multiple layers. It would still probably taste fine, though.

Making spaghetti squash lasagna boats:

So, the heart of this recipe and here is how you can make it. The steps to make spaghetti squash lasagna boats are very simple. You can prepare multiple layers at same time to save your time.

- ➤ First of all roast the spaghetti squash in the oven. You can use higher temperature to do it faster.
- ➤ Let it roast and sauté garlic in olive oil with salt and pepper until brown in a pan meanwhile. Then add marinara sauce or any other seasoning you like in it and mix them together.

> - Stir together the parmesan, ricotta and olive oil in a bowl. Keep enough room so that you may add spaghetti squash into it later.
> - Finally, all that's left is the assembly of your stuffed spaghetti squash lasagna. To start, mix the squash strands into the bowl with the cheeses.
> - Now, just alternate the layers inside the empty shells – spaghetti squash, marinara, and mozzarella. You can do just one layer of each to keep it simple or multiple thin layers if you want that layered aspect of lasagna.

Place the assembled spaghetti squash lasagna boats into the oven to melt the cheese. It's up to you how much you want it to brown. Sprinkle with a little parsley at the end for color, but that's totally optional.

There you go – easy, low carb lasagna stuffed spaghetti squash!

Nutrition:

287 kcal | 22g fat | 14g protein | 10g carbs

Ingredients:

- Spaghetti squash – 1 medium
- Olive oil – 4 tsp
- Marinara sauce – ½ cup
- Italian seasoning – 1 tsp
- Ricotta cheese – 2/3 cheeses
- Grated parmesan cheese – 1/3 cup
- Mozzarella cheese – 2/3 cup
- Salt and pepper to taste

Instructions:

- Preheat the oven to 425°F/218°C and roast spaghetti squash in it.
- Take a bowl and mix together ricotta cheese, parmesan cheese and olive oil. Keep enough room to add spaghetti squash in it later.
- When spaghetti squash is ready, take it out of the oven but don't turn off the oven and keep it at 425°F
- Cut the squash in half lengthwise. Place open side up onto the baking pan and use a fork to release strands.
- Transfer the spaghetti squash strands into the large bowl with the ricotta and parmesan cheeses. Mix together. Season with sea salt to taste.
- Stuff the spaghetti squash mixture back into the empty shells on the baking pan. Top with marinara mixture. Sprinkle shredded mozzarella on top. (If desired, you can create several thinner layers of each mixture)
- Return the lasagna spaghetti squash boats to the oven for about 10 minutes, until the cheese melts.
- Here are your low carb boats ready to take you into the ocean of taste!

Note:

- Do not turn off the oven after taking spaghetti squash out of it and save your time.
- Use marinara sauce, it will surely add a lot of taste.

5- <u>Ketogenic vegan Sushi Bowl</u>

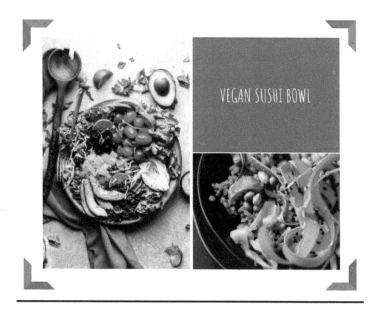

A magical combination of cucumber, avocado and nori that is keto friendly and vegan friendly is going to make you forget any other combination. An unmatchable dinner that is deliciously ketogenic and is going to bring fun in your keto diet schedule.

Finding this dish in both formats i.e. ketogenic & vegetarian is bit challenging task. You may find a recipe that is ketogenic but is not vegetarian as it may include salmon fish or meat. If you find a vegetarian recipe than it may have rice in it that makes it high carb and hence is not ketogenic. So, you are going to make a combination of vegetarian and ketogenic dishes into one bowl and that bowl is "Ketogenic vegan Sushi bowl".

Traditionally, if you buy a vegetarian sushi bowl from a restaurant, it will mostly contain rice rolls and you cannot ignore the presence of rice if you are following a ketogenic diet. In this recipe we are going to replace rice with another substitute that is going to retain the taste of this dish as well. There's no rolling involved, which means they're much easier to make. You can get more creative with toppings, too, since you aren't limited to options that roll up well. Best of all, these fresh but hearty bowls keep me fueled for hours.

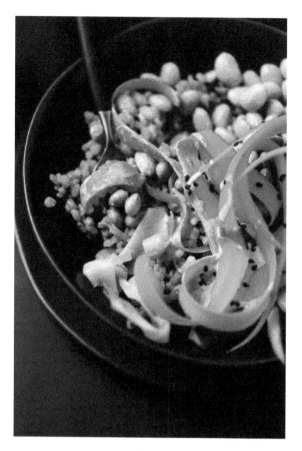

There is a whole universe of spices and variations that you can add into this dish according to your choice. But yes, if you add spicy mayo sauce on top, ohhh, that is the real kicker! I will transform your "Keto healthy bowl" into a "Magical tasty bowl". You can try other variations as well. These variations can take your dish to another level!

Some useful tips:

These are some tips that you may like to consider in order to enhance taste of your dish.

- ➤ Try to use homemade salad recipe even if you can buy one from store.
- ➤ You can add vegetables like bell pepper, asparagus, carrots, zucchini and summer squash and they will surely bring a healthier taste to your dish.
- ➤ For proteins, it is better that you use tofu (It will keep your dish soy-free) or you may also use homemade vegan lox.
- ➤ If tofu or lox are not available, you can use toona as well.

Nutrition:

596 kcal | 25g fat | 16.5g proteins | 4g carbs

Ingredients:

- Cooked cauliflower rice – ½ cup
- Homemade seaweed salad – 26g
- Cucumber slices – ¼ cup
- Vegan toona or protein of your choice – 1/3 cup

Toppings:

- Avocado sliced – 34g
- Sesame seeds – 1 tsp
- Micro greens – 1 tsp

Instructions:

- Take all the vegans and cut them in slices or cubes as you like.

- Take a bowl and add cauliflower along with toona and homemade seaweed salad. Mix them with your favorite spices.
- If you don't want anything spicy you can just skip this step.
- Now add other ingredients into the bowl and dress them according to your liking and serve.

Note:

You can use any protein of your choice instead of toona or tofu.

Ketogenic Dessert recipes

How the life is possible without dessert. Dessert is one of the biggest need of the body after oxygen (just kidding ;-)). Even one who is following a diet plan wishes to have some dessert that may not ruin his diet and also fulfil his taste bud's requirements. So keeping in view all this things and keto requirements, few recipes are here for you to enjoy desert in your keto diet plan to make your keto diet a real fun for you. So, let's get started!'

1- <u>Ketogenic chocolate mug cake</u>

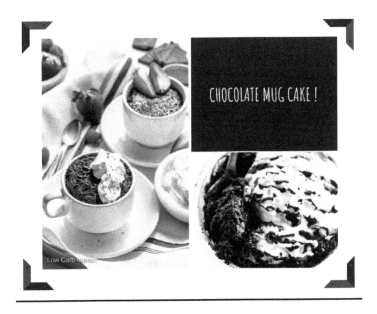

A cup that has absorbed whole world into it, made with almond flour and cocoa giving it a perfect cake texture is the perfect dessert recipe for you during your keto days.

This cake is different:

Most of the mug cakes use whole egg. Yes, it's true that whole egg is efficient but it also makes cakes really dense and tough. And we want to give you something really soft and moist. So there is a hack that you can use. Just use egg yolk and mayonnaise. The yolk adds structure to the cake and the mayo makes it nice and moist.

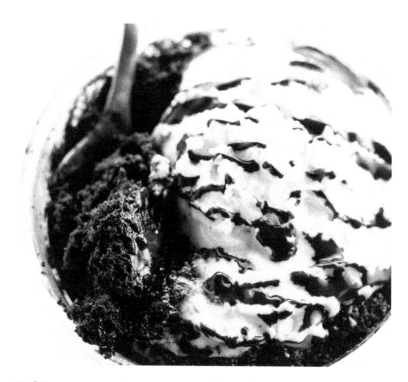

Taking your cake to a next level:

If you really want to satisfy your taste buds. Then you must try variations with your cake. There are some tips that you may like to consider.

- ➢ Try a different taste by adding some berries into the batter
- ➢ You can also add a few teaspoon flavoring extract like vanilla extract etc. to the batter
- ➢ Put a spoon of sugar-free jelly as topping over your cake, yummy!!
- ➢ Put a small square of dark chocolate in the middle of the batter before cooking.
- ➢ Top with sugar-free homemade hot fudge or store bought sugar-free chocolate sauce
- ➢ Top with whipped cream or whipped coconut cream
- ➢ Sprinkle cinnamon, cocoa powder, powdered sweetener or grated chocolate on top

What to do with the leftover egg white:

As you will be using just egg yolk in making and you have got leftover egg white and you don't know what to do with it. You have got options to do. Refrigerate it if you don't want to use it in recipe at all. But if you have got plans to use it, then you can use it in making homemade mayonnaise, whip it and make cream cheese clouds. Or you can save it to make another mug cake afterwards. Or fry the egg white in your morning eggs!

Adding peanut butter (Optional):

When it comes to adding extras to your cake, you have got a lot options to try. One of the recommended extras is peanut butter. Melt butter in microwave, add almond flour or coconut flour, sweetener of your choice, cocoa powder, baking powder, vanilla and beaten eggs. Whisk them well and microwave for about 60 seconds. Don't over-cook it otherwise it will become dry. Once ready, serve it with your cup cake.

Nutrition:

272 kcal | 7g carbs | 9g proteins | 23g fats

Ingredients:

- Almond flour – 2tsp
- Cocoa powder – 1 tsp
- Swerve or lakanto (or any other low-carb sugar) – 1tsp
- Baking powder – ¼ tsp
- Mayonnaise – 1 tsp
- 1 large egg yolk
- Water – 1tsp

Instructions:

- Fluff up the almond flour with a whisk before measuring and SIFT THE COCOA POWDER BEFORE MEASURING. (I sift any cocoa powder I buy and keep it in an air-tight container. This breaks apart any lumps for more accurate measuring. Using compacted cocoa results in using more cocoa and a bitter cake.)

Method:

- Measure the dry ingredients into a mug or jelly jar and mix completely with a fork.

- Add the mayonnaise, egg yolk, and water, stirring completely making sure to get it all from the bottom. Let batter sit 1-2 minutes.
- Microwave for 50 seconds, depending on your microwave. 3 Net Carbs.

2- <u>Ketogenic ice cream</u>

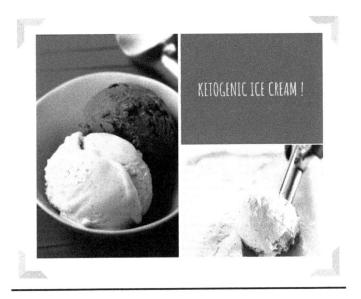

A ketogenic dairy-free and low carb ice cream that not only keto followers will enjoy but also those who are not following any diet will fall in love with it. Creamy smooth ice cream without sugar in it is an ultimate dessert for keto diet followers.

The thing that makes this ice cream keto friendly is the sugar-free condensed milk that is sweetened with sweeteners. Most of the ice creams are not ketogenic because of added milk and sugar. Ketogenic ice creams are also available in stores nowadays but making ice cream at home with your own hands gives an exceptional taste.

As a keto diet follower you are not allowed to eat ice cream. But this recipe is an ultimate resolve for you if you are an ice cream lover. A very simple recipe and you will have your ice cream without harming your diet plan.

Making condensed milk:

As you need a keto ice cream so you will need condensed milk. Here is the procedure of making it.

➢ Take a sauce pan and melt butter in it. Ad heavy cream and powdered sweetener of your choice and then simmer for a long time to reduce. Wait until the liquid evaporates and mixture becomes thick forming condensed milk.

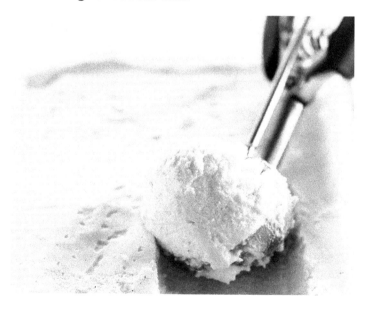

Using ice cream maker:

It is possible to make ice cream without an ice cream maker but still it is recommended that you use ice cream maker as it makes it much easier to make this recipe. It will also help in making recipe a lot consistent.

If you've got one, just pour ice cream mixture into it and let it churn until it becomes thick and soft like ice cream. It will take about 20-25 minutes. After churning, place the ice cream into container of your choice and freeze for few hours to get more firm keto friendly ice cream.

If you use ice cream maker then you will not need MCT oil or powder. If you want to make it without ice cream maker, you must include MCT oil.

Toppings and extras:

Adding vanilla extract into your ice cream will simply make it tastier and give it an enhanced flavor. Following are some topping options that you may like to consider before freezing your ice cream:

- Berries including blue berries, raspberries or strawberries
- Sugar-free chocolate chips or wafers
- Caramel sauce (Sugar free)
- Chunks of chocolate chip cookies.

Storing for future use:

You can store this ice cream like any other ice cream in a freezer. But it may harden a little more than normal ice cream as we don't have some artificial ingredients added into it. If it hardens too much, let it rest for a while in room temperature until soft.

Nutrition:

347 kcal | 36g fats | 2g proteins |3g carbs

Ingredients:

- Divided heavy cream – 4 cups
- Vanilla extract – 1 tsp
- Butter – 3 tsp
- Sweetener of your choice (powdered) – 1/3 cup
- MCT oil – ¼ cup (optional)
- Vanilla bean (optional) – 1 medium

Instructions:

- Take a large bottom sauce pan and put over heat. Add butter and half of the heavy cream along with sweetener into it and let boil until reduced. Then simmer for 30-45 minutes and stir occasionally until the mixture becomes thick. Check if the mixture is reduced to half it means it is ready.
- Add a bowl and pour the thick mixture into it. Allow the mixture to cool at room temperature.
- Now add vanilla extract, vanilla beans and whisk with MCT oil. (Optional)
- Now add the remaining 2 cups of heavy cream into the bowl containing mixture. Let it smooth.
- Add the mixture into ice cream maker and churn until thick like ice cream.
- Top the ice cream with your favorite berries.

- Now chill the mixture in the fridge for about 3-4 hours for best results. You can also skip this step if you don't have much time.

Note:

- If you don't want to use heavy cream you can use coconut milk or almond milk instead.

3- <u>Keto peanut chocolate blocks</u>

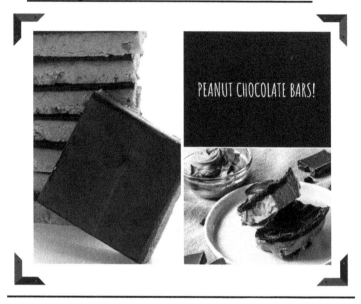

No sugar, no carbs, no dairy! This recipe is going to be one of the best things you have ever experienced. Low carb and high fat peanut butter bars will make a delicious ketogenic dessert that will be a fat bomb and it also tastes like a normal delicious chocolate. Beauty of dish is that it is not only for followers of keto diet but is also for those who have never followed any kind of diet. Peanut butter makes a delicious mouthwatering combination with creamy chocolate. In no time, this recipe can be prepared but the taste cannot be forgotten whole life.

<u>Is peanut butter suitable in keto?</u>

So, many people will not consider peanut butter during keto diet as peanuts are technically legumes and can cause inflammation in the body. Yet there are people who have been enjoying peanuts during their diet without any health problems. Naturally, peanut butter is low carb and contains high fats but make sure to look for sugar-free peanut butter while buying as there are some brands which contain added sugar in them. You can justify peanuts but can never justify sugar when you are living ketogenically!

Ingredients for no bake peanut butter bars:

- ➤ Make sure you buy sugar-free peanut butter. Crunchy peanut butter will be a lot tasty if you consider but it is your choice. You may like to add smooth butter. Do as you like.
- ➤ Also use butter and coconut flour. Butter will bind the ingredients together and coconut flour will give the bars structure.
- ➤ Instead of sugar, always use keto friendly sweetener when you are following keto diet. In this recipe, it is preferred to use powdered sweetener instead of liquid.
- ➤ You can make smooth chocolate bar by melting sugar-free lily's milk chocolate bar.

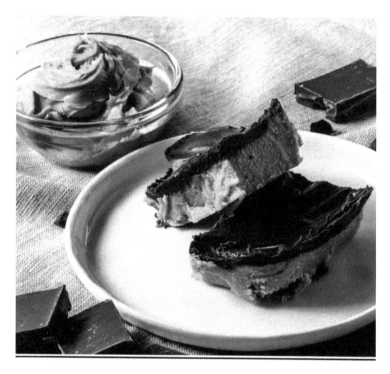

Important step: To make the creamy peanut butter layer, mix natural peanut butter, coconut flour, and Lakanto Powdered Sweetener. I loved the added texture that crunchy peanut butter added to the No-Bake Keto Peanut Butter Chocolate Bars, but you can use creamy if you prefer.

Tip: You can use almond flour in place of coconut flour. The conversion is 1/4 cup coconut flour is equal to 1 cup of almond flour.

Alternative for peanut butter:

If you find it risky to use peanut butter in keto diet, no worries! Use almond butter instead. But make sure it is sugar-free and is natural nut butter.

Melting chocolate without hardening:

If you want to keep the chocolate soft and avoid any hardening, then microwave the chocolate in low settings so it may melt slowly. Once chocolate is melt, you have options whether you want to make chocolate bars or chocolate cups!

Nutrition:

150kcal | 5g carbs | 4g proteins | 13g fats

Ingredients:

- Peanut butter – 1 cup
- Softened butter – 4 tsp
- Powdered sweetener – 2/3 cup
- Coconut flour – 2 tsp
- Butter (for topping) – 1 tsp
- Lily's cream milk chocolate – 1-3 oz

Instructions:

- Take a bowl and add butter in it. Beat the butter at high speed to soften it.
- Add powdered sweetener of your choice, peanut butter and coconut flour in the softened butter and beat again at medium speed and make sure to mix all the ingredients thoroughly.
- Take a baking pan and line it with parchment paper or grease it with oil or butter. Spread the peanut butter evenly over the pan and place in freezer for about 10-15 minutes.

- Take a glass container and add lily's smooth chocolate bar in it with butter and microwave for 30 seconds on low power until melted. Make sure to stir it in intervals.
- Remove the baking pan from freezer and pour the melted chocolate over peanut layer evenly.
- Again place the pan in the freezer for few hours until the bars are set. Once they have setup, you can store in freezer or fridge.
- Here is your peanut butter chocolate ready to please you.

Note:

- Do not cook the chocolate too much otherwise it will become hard.
- Make sure to use sugar-free peanut butter or almond butter.

4- Low- carb walnut snow balls

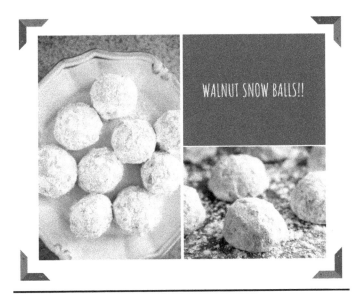

Mexican wedding cookies, Russian tea cakes, Italian wedding cookies call this dish with any name yet the taste is the iconic that will show the magic in with any name used to call it!

A low carb dessert with an unmatchable taste and crunch will be one of "Must have" recipes for you during your keto diet.

Difference between Mexican and Italian snow balls:

These walnut snow balls are enjoyed in all countries of the world ranging from Spain and Italy in Europe to Mexico and Russia in America and Asia! Every country has its own variation for this recipe. The basic different although is the choice of nuts. Every country is 'NUTS' specific in making this recipe. You can also add nuts according to your choice or your country's choice, yet this recipe includes walnut as the main ingredient.

Which flour to use, coconut or almond?

Coconut flour works best in this recipe. Almond flour is so far not found to fit as ingredient in this recipe so it's not recommended to use almond flour. The thing that makes coconut flour more preferable in this recipe is that it is more powder like which helps to make keto snowballs that melt in your mouth.

Moreover, almond flour is less absorbent and hence you require more flour to make the same keto recipe that you can make by using lesser coconut flour. If you want to make this recipe with almond flour, you will need three times more almond flour than that of coconut flour.

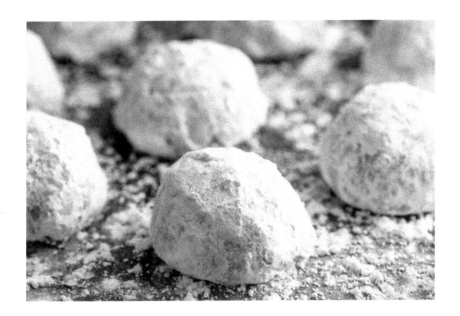

How to sweeten the snowballs?

Okay! So one thing is for sure that we are not going to use sugar as sweetener as it can ruin your keto diet. So you will use any artificial sugar-free sweetener of your choice. Recommended sweetener is 'Confection Erythritol'. It is a low carb sweetener and is easily available in stores. You can also use homemade sweetener as well. It depends on your choice.

Using walnuts in this recipe:

Walnuts have got one of the best profiles to be used as NUT in this great dessert recipe. You can also use walnut flour or walnut spiced cookies in this recipe as well. You can make walnut flour by processing walnuts in a food process in few spins. You can add this flour in any dessert recipe or salad during your keto diet.

Nutrition:

127 kcal | 12g fats | 3g carbs | 2g proteins

Ingredients:

- Walnuts – 1 cup
- Coconut flour – ½ cup
- Melted butter – ½ cup
- 1 Large egg
- Vanilla extract – ½ tsp
- Liquid stevia – 50-52 drops
- Swerve confectioner – ½ cup

Instructions:

- Take a bowl and add melted butter, egg, stevia and vanilla extract in it and whisk.
- Take another bowl and coconut flour into it along with ¼ cup swerve. Ground walnuts in a food processor and add the =ground walnuts into the coconut flour mixture.
- In two parts, add dry mixture to the wet and whisk to combine. At this point the dough should be soft but firm enough to form into balls by hand without it sticking to your palms. If it is not the right consistency add 1 to 2 tablespoons of additional coconut flour and combine.
- Pre heat the oven to 300 °F and line the baking sheet with parchment paper.

- Make 15 to 17 equal balls and place them on baking sheet. Make sure that they do not spread in oven. Bake for about 30-35 minutes.
- Take the baking sheet out and let the balls cool for 5 minutes. Then roll the balls in remaining ¼ cup swerve.
- Place the balls back on the parchment paper and allow cooling fully before eating. Here are your crunchy Walnut snow balls! Enjoy the taste!

Note:

It is not recommended to use almond flour in this recipe.

5- <u>Ketogenic brownies</u>

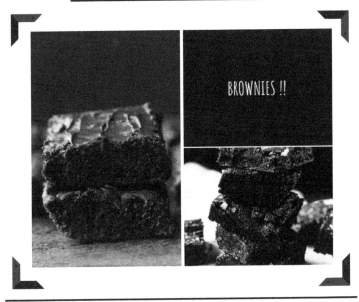

The best and easiest low carb keto brownies. Even people who aren't on a keto diet will love these unbelievably fudgy chocolate brownies! These impossibly fudgy chocolate brownies are almost guaranteed to win you over.

It's one of those must-try recipes, because you really need to try them at least once in your life to discover how shockingly good they are!

The simple recipe is so rich and delicious; you might never go back to boxed brownies again. Feel free to stir a handful of chopped pecans, almonds, or walnuts into the batter. Or throw in some shredded coconut, cacao nibs, or chocolate chips.

To come up with this recipe, I simply adapted my keto chocolate cake into brownies.

Since I know brownies have more fat, less flour, and less leavening than cake, I changed the ingredient proportions accordingly.

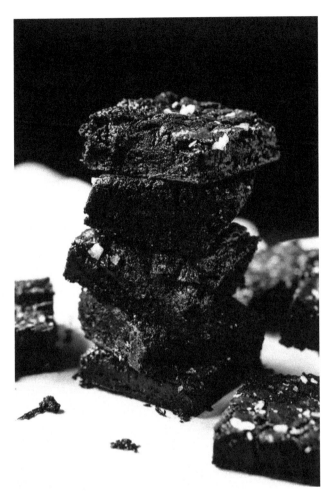

The first try wasn't perfect, but recipe experiments are seldom perfect on the first try, and I quite enjoyed eating the fall-apart-gooey flourless homemade brownie rejects.

The moist chocolate brownies can be made with either regular sugar (for non keto) or granulated erythritol. If making them keto, be sure to buy granulated erythritol, not powdered. Or for paleo brownies, you can also use coconut sugar.

Moist, chewy and fudgy on the inside with a crisp crinkle layer on the top making these the world's BEST keto brownies. They're rich and delicious and will satisfy your chocolate cravings with just 1 net carb per brownie!

Almond flour works great for keto desserts and is my favorite option and I highly recommend sticking with it. If you'd prefer to use coconut flour, I suggest substituting 1/4 the amount of almond flour with coconut flour. For example, this recipe calls for 1/2 cup almond flour so about 2 tablespoons coconut flour should be enough.

Nutrition:

116 kcal | 3g carbs | 2g proteins | 5g Fats

Ingredients:

- Almond flour – 1 cup
- Cocoa powder – ¼ cup
- Regular cocoa or Dutch cocoa – 2 tsp
- Baking powder – 1 tsp
- Salt – ½ tsp
- Melted coconut oil or butter – 1/3 cup
- Water – 3 tsp
- 2 Eggs
- Erythritol – 2/3 cup
- Vanilla extract – 1 tsp

Instructions:

- Pre heat oven to 350°F or 175°C and line baking pan with parchment paper or grease with butter.

- Take a bowl and add almond flour, cocoa powder. Baking powder. Erythritol and coffee into it. Whisk all ingredients well.
- Melt butter and chocolate for about 30 seconds until melted in an oven. Add eggs and vanilla into it and gently whisk them together. Do not over mix otherwise the batter will become cake like.
- Now pour the batter onto a the baking sheet and bake for around 18-20 minutes. When baked, let it cool for 30 minutes or more in the fridge and slice into small square pieces and enjoy the dish heartily!

Note:

Do not over bake the batter. If the batter looks giggly, remove it from the oven after 25 minutes and it will set at room temperature. It is normal to see butter pooling on top the brownies.

Closing Notes

Hope you have tasted all the recipes and have made a new list of your favorite meals. It happens, after following ketogenic diet, your list of favorite meals changes. Now you have one more responsibility. Don't consider this book as just a single cook book; it can save someone's life if taken seriously. So keep sharing as sharing is caring!

Author,

Antonio Tagliafierro

CPSIA information can be obtained
at www.ICGtesting.com
Printed in the USA
BVHW021554220221
600777BV00010B/524